Hygiene and Health in Developing Countries - Recent Advances

Edited by Sonja Šostar Turk and Urška Rozman

Published in London, United Kingdom

Hygiene and Health in Developing Countries - Recent Advances
http://dx.doi.org/10.5772/intechopen.100959
Edited by Sonja Šostar Turk and Urška Rozman

Contributors
Tigist Gashaw, Abera Jambo, Nadzeya Dziarzhynskaya, Larisa Hindziuk, Andrey Hindziuk, Victor Dang Mvongo, Paul Blaise Mabou, Célestin Defo, Paul Fabrice Nguema, Anil Kumar Mishra, Auguste Ombolo, Jude Robinson, Hamilton Majiwa, Olivia Howland, Fhumulani M. Mulaudzi, Nombulelo V. Sepeng, Ndivhaleni R. Lavhelani, Tintswalo V. Nesengane

First published in London, United Kingdom, 2022 by IntechOpen
IntechOpen is the global imprint of INTECHOPEN LIMITED, registered in England and Wales, registration number: 11086078, 5 Princes Gate Court, London, SW7 2QJ, United Kingdom

British Library Cataloguing-in-Publication Data
A catalogue record for this book is available from the British Library

Additional hard and PDF copies can be obtained from orders@intechopen.com

Hygiene and Health in Developing Countries - Recent Advances
Edited by Sonja Šostar Turk and Urška Rozman
p. cm.
Print ISBN 978-1-80356-623-8
Online ISBN 978-1-80356-624-5
eBook (PDF) ISBN 978-1-80356-625-2

Meet the editors

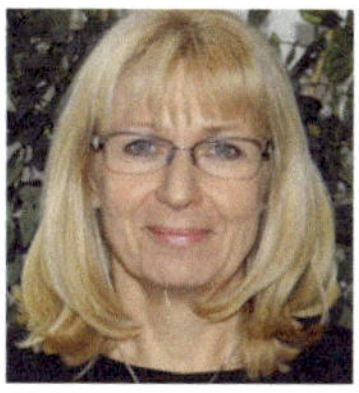

Prof. Sonja Šostar Turk, Ph.D., is a Professor of Textile Chemistry and Environmental Engineering at the University of Maribor, Slovenia. Since 2008 she has been employed at the Faculty of Health Sciences at the same university where she is Vice-Dean for Postgraduate Studies, head of the Department of Interdisciplinary Sciences, and head of the Institute of Balneology and Climatology. She is a lecturer and co-lecturer of several courses in nursing, management in health and social organization, and food safety. Her research focuses on environmental health, hospital hygiene, and food safety. She has coordinated ten European projects and led forty-one basic and applied national projects and fifteen bilateral projects. She has one patent to her credit. In 2014, she received the prestigious United Nations National Energy Globe Award 2014 in the "Water" category for a project with the acronym SMILES under the 7th EU Framework Program (FP7).

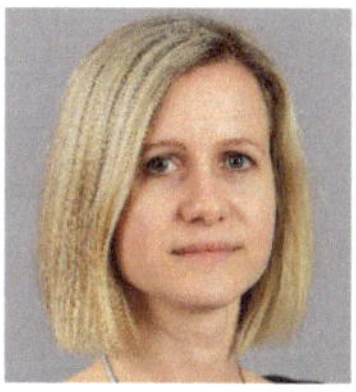

Assist. Prof. Urška Rozman, Ph.D., is an Assistant Professor of Biology at the University of Maribor, Slovenia. She obtained her master's degree in Biology and her Ph.D. in Ecological Sciences from the same university. She participates in courses in nursing, management in health and social organization, and food safety. She has been involved in several European and national projects in environmental health, hospital hygiene, and food safety. For the last three years, she has participated in the National Program on Nutrition and Physical Activity for Health 2015–2025, a project of the Ministry of Health.

Contents

Preface IX

Chapter 1 1
Understanding Household Water Hygiene in Resource-Limited Settings in Kenya
by Jude Robinson, Hamilton Majiwa and Olivia Howland

Chapter 2 17
Perspective Chapter: Access to Rural Water and Sanitation Services in Cameroon within the Context of Sustainable Development Goals (SDGs)
by Victor Dang Mvongo, Paul Blaise Mabou, Célestin Defo, Paul Fabrice Nguema, Anil Kumar Mishra and Auguste Ombolo

Chapter 3 31
Typhoid in Less Developed Countries: A Major Public Health Concern
by Tigist Gashaw and Abera Jambo

Chapter 4 45
Maintaining Hand Hygiene in the Informal Settlements: Reflections on Compliance for Covid-19 Preventative Measures
by Fhumulani M. Mulaudzi, Nombulelo V. Sepeng, Ndivhaleni R. Lavhelani and Tintswalo V. Nesengani

Chapter 5 57
Air Pollution Monitoring and Its Health Impact in Belarus
by Nadzeya Dziarzhynskaya, Larisa Hindziuk and Andrey Hindziuk

Preface

In developing countries, climate change means that many more people find themselves living in areas of environmental disadvantage, with water insecurity recognized as a major challenge to health. Water is a global resource recognized by the United Nations in its Sustainable Development Goals (SDG); SDG 6 is "clean water and sanitation for all." Global water insecurity in the context of climate change has negative effects on hygiene, food security, and people's physical and mental health. Especially in rural areas, different factors are contributing to poor access to water and sanitation services such as the poor application of the policy and legal framework for rural water and sanitation services management, the poor coordination of interventions between the actors involved in the sector, the low financial viability of rural water and sanitation services management, the low efficiency of expenditure related to water and sanitation, and the lack of human resources in the sector. One of the major public health concerns in less developed countries with impoverished areas with unsafe drinking water sources and poor sanitation, connected to contaminated food and water, remains typhoid fever. Inadequate water supplies and sanitation measures may also cause illnesses like diarrhea. It is necessary to recognize how human wellbeing is significantly dependent on safe drinking water, sanitation, and hygiene. A lack of running water and poor sanitation also affects community members' compliance with Covid-19 preventive measures.

The editors of this volume are experts in the field of environmental health, hygiene, and food safety. As such, this book provides readers with an understanding of the importance of climate change as it relates to the safety of drinking water and food as well as hygiene, especially in developing countries. The editors are thankful to all authors who have included their work in this book.

Dr. Sonja Šostar Turk, Ph.D.
Professor,
Faculty of Health Sciences,
University of Maribor,
Maribor, Slovenia

Dr. Urška Rozman, Ph.D.
Assistant Professor,
Faculty of Health Sciences,
University of Maribor,
Maribor, Slovenia

Chapter 1

Understanding Household Water Hygiene in Resource-Limited Settings in Kenya

Jude Robinson, Hamilton Majiwa and Olivia Howland

Abstract

Climate change means that many more people find themselves living in areas of environmental disadvantage, with water insecurity recognized as a major health issue. Local ecologies shape everyday hygiene practices in households as people respond to diurnal and seasonal changes in their external environment. Periods of water shortage paradoxically increase the risk of waterborne diseases such as cholera, exacerbated by reduced washing to conserve limited supplies. Unpredictable periods of drought and/or flooding compromise household income, and families cannot afford the basic resources they need to keep themselves and others clean. The risks of water borne diseases, such as typhoid, giardia and cholera, are reduced by strategies that improve the sourcing, storage, and treatment of drinking water in areas of environmental disadvantage. In this chapter we first outline global water insecurity in the context of climate change and the negative effects on people's physical and mental health. We develop our ideas by drawing on our fieldwork, specifically depth interviews with over 50 people living in Kware, Ongata Rongai outside Nairobi, Kenya, to consider how people negotiate persistent water insecurity in resource-limited settings. We conclude the chapter with reflections on the barriers and opportunities to improve water security and hygiene practices.

Keywords: water insecurity, everyday hygiene, health inequalities, water quality, climate change, poverty, gender

1. Introduction

The effects of climate change are already being felt everywhere and outstandingly, they are felt through water. According to UNICEF there is increased demand for water: low rainfall causes drought, and heavy rainfall and flooding can damage water sources and sanitation facilities, often carrying runoff and waste into streams and lakes and so contaminating the water supply. Climate change means that many more people find themselves living in areas of environmental disadvantage, with water insecurity is recognized as a major challenge to health [1]. Water is a global resource, recognized by the United Nations in their Sustainable Development Goals (SDGs) as Clean Water and Sanitation (SDG 6); with the hazards relating to changing patterns of rainfall and rising temperatures crucial to Life on Land (SDG 15) and Life Below Water (SDG 14) as priorities for humans to achieve a sustainable future [2]. While people living in some areas of the world have suffered historically from long term water scarcity and/or periodic flooding, it is estimated that by 2030, around half the world's population will experience water insecurity [3]. Despite investments in infrastructure to store and conserve water, in recent decades areas of Europe, US, Africa, Asia and Australia have been adversely affected by changing rainfall patterns, leading to water insecurity and altered social and physical environments [4].

Here, we consider global water insecurity in the context of climate change and the negative effects that access to too much or too little water has on hygiene and on people's physical and mental health. Water insecurity is exacerbated by climate change, with elevated temperatures and unpredictable patterns of rainfall. High temperatures, lack of cloud cover and decreased rainfall lead to periods of drought, associated with an increased risk of subsequent catastrophic events, such as fires [5], dust storms [6] or the erosion of deforested and/or degraded land when rain eventually falls [7]. Drought leads to pressures on sites where water is found and there are tensions and conflicts between people and organizations who need to access water for drinking, hygiene, washing, industries and agriculture [8]. Episodes of extreme precipitation and flood events due to climate change contribute to lower temperatures, flooding and further environmental degradation [9]. These devastating effects are experienced by animals as well as people as they destroy landscapes and habitats [10], as well as settlements and wider infrastructure such as roads, bridges and sanitation systems [11]. Water insecurity and associated environmental degradation has adversely impacted on food security, leading to failure of successive harvests and the death of livestock, leading to long-term shifts in livelihoods as well as impacting on national economies [12].

Globally, there is enough fresh water for the current human and animal population, however it is unevenly distributed across regions and countries and other human actions contribute to its scarcity. Non-climatic events, such as human war and conflict destroy water infrastructures and/or reduce access to water sources and contribute directly to the forced migrations of people and livestock, which in turn place stress on the water supplies in the areas that they move to [13]. Water supplies are further compromised by historic and ongoing contamination from industry and agriculture, who are intensive extractors of water supplies [4]. Inequalities in water availability are compounded by poor water management, the over extraction of ground water driven by increased consumption and global population increases [14]. Population increases are highest in areas of the Global South where water is often a scare resource, but there are other socio-political factors that need to be considered as elites in the Global South do not suffer from the effects of water insecurity. An analysis of Day Zero, the recent water crisis in Cape Town, South Africa (2015–2017) suggests that contributing factors to differing patterns of water consumption were both racialized and classed, with white urban elites less affected by long term water shortages [15]. In addition, Black South Africans living in the poorest areas of Cape Town had suffered persistent water scarcity prior to 2015. Similarly evidence from the US and Canada found racial and geographic inequalities between the quality and affordability of water supplies between those classed as rich and poor in the Global North, debunking what they term the 'myths of household water insecurity' [16]. Deitz and Meehan [17] identify a lack of investment in water infrastructure, what they term 'plumbing poverty', as the reason why the poorest people in the US cannot always access clean water.

People require a minimum of 20–50 liters of clean water a day to meet their basic needs, and around 2 liters needs to be suitable for drinking, although the amount depends on the person and the context [18]. While those in the Global North may use over 150 liters of water a day for washing, cleaning, cooking, drinking and flushing, other people, many of whom live in the Global South, have access to less than 20 liters of water per day. While access to piped water has increased globally between 2000 and 2017, it remains lowest in countries in sub-Saharan Africa and tends to be concentrated in urban rather than rural areas [19]. Disease and infection relate to water quality as well as water quantity, and van Vliet et al. [20] advocate the treatment of waste water as a vital means of increasing the availability and safety of water. There is emerging evidence that pathogens respond to increased temperatures and higher incidences of enteric (intestinal) infections are found in water as temperatures rise [21]. Periods of water shortage paradoxically lead to increased rates of waterborne diseases such as cholera, as pressure on water compromises choices of water sources and hygiene practices, and associated food shortages increases vulnerability to disease. Even short periods of drought may force people to migrate and congregate in areas lacking basic sanitary infrastructure [22]. There is evidence of gendered inequalities in terms of water access, with men better able to access water compared to women in the same communities and households [23]. Gendered and other intersectional inequalities persist within resources-limited communities, with pregnant women and children particularly vulnerable to the effects of drought [24, 25].

Climate change and water insecurity affect mental and well as physical health [26]. Periods of drought or flooding, and associated shifts in ecologies and loss of livelihood are associated with depression and anxiety for men and women [27]. The pressure on livelihood linked to water insecurity can mean that men need to leave their homes to look for work in urban areas or in other countries. This occupational migration puts undue pressure on the remaining household members, who take on additional roles and responsibilities and suffer from reduced opportunities [28]. Younger people may have to leave school to contribute their labor to the household or in local employment, with long term consequences for their future physical and mental health [29]. Migrant workers also suffer from poor mental health, associated with a loss of status, support and community, and they often engage in risky health practices such as drinking alcohol, taking drugs and gambling [30, 31]. Lacking access to the resources needed maintain a good personal appearance can impact on mental health and wellbeing [32]. Having access to water to wash clothes and bodies is essential for personal cleanliness, and personal hygiene is compromised by water insecurity when water for drinking and cooking is prioritized over other uses. Looking and feeling 'dirty' leads to social and physical exclusion from many areas of communal life necessary for social standing and personal dignity [33]. In these ways water insecurity affects individuals, household and communities.

2. Everyday clean/Usafi Kila Siku

We developed *Everyday Clean/ Usafi Kila Siku* to explore practices of health and hygiene in resource-limited settings in Kenya. Our research was funded by *HORN—One Health Network for the Horn of Africa*, and international partnership funded through the United Kingdom Research and Innovation (UKRI) Global Challenges Research Fund (GCRF) scheme. Our study was designed to understand how washing practices in low-income settings are mediated by social, economic and physical environments and to further understand the strategies people have developed to mitigate any perceived risks to their health. While the research took place across three sites, here we draw on our research with 53 participants living in the peri-urban, low-income community of Kware in Ongata Rongai, on the outer edge of the city of Nairobi, in Kajiado County. We applied for ethical approval through the International Livestock Research Institute in Kenya, gained additional approval from the University of Liverpool, UK, and registered the project with the National Commission for Science Technology and Innovation (NACOSTI) in Kenya.

Kware is an informal settlement, 17 miles south of the centre of Nairobi and close to the eastern edge of the Nairobi National Park. There were a recorded 29,000 residents in the wider area of Ongata Rongai in the 2009 Census, which is now thought to have grown to around 40,000 residents in 2019. The area is ethnically diverse, and as well as the original Maasai, there are people who identify as Boran, Kalenjin, Kikuyu, Kamba, Kisii, Luhya and Luo. While people have settled on the old quarry site (Kware) since the 1960's, the original settlers were surrounded by green space and were able to keep livestock and get water from the nearby Mbagathi river. Over the last 10–15 years the rapid population growth has led to an expansion of informal housing, a reduction of green space and trees, with little additional infrastructure in terms of roads, services such as waste collection and drainage. Some houses do not have electricity, although others access generators and electricity supplies. Charcoal is the main fuel used for cooking and boiling water. Around 4–8 households share pit latrines within each compound, which overflow when flooded, and open defecation is a problem for the community. Water is accessed via boreholes where people can take their containers to buy water at between United States Dollars (USD) 0.20 to USD 0.50 for 20 liters, depending on availability, from water vendors who carry containers or use donkey carts to bring water to the community, and water tankers who bring water to stands on the main roads that run through Ongata Rongai. Some people collect water from the Mbagathi river, and from the smaller streams that flow in drainage ditches during the rainy season. Water is stored in large, repurposed plastic containers of 10–20 liters with handles (often termed 'jerrycans') outside and inside people's homes and transferred to smaller containers for use. There is limited waste (rubbish) collection from the settlement, and many people dump discarded items, which are then burned in situ.

2.1 Methods

Prior to starting the research late in 2019, we consulted with representatives from Kware, who were strongly supportive of the need for the study and approved of our responsive and exploratory study design. It was through these initial discussions that we recognized the critical important of water access, water quality and pricing to people living on low income, and these issues were added to the interview guide for the study. The research was originally planned in two phases, but this was extended to three phases due to the pandemic and the need to collect further data as new themes emerged from our ongoing analysis. The interview guide used for the first phase of data collection (P1) in December 2019 included questions on the resources needed for the washing of bodies, the washing of clothes and linen and general household hygiene issues, such as food hygiene and any occupational issues. We continued these lines of inquiry during the second phase of interviews (P2) in September 2021 and explored any changing hygiene practices and water access due to the ongoing COVID-19 pandemic. For the final phase of interviews in March 2022 (P3), we explored issues of trust around water supplies and issues of water security. As we are all trained anthropologists, we used inductive and exploratory methods throughout and adapted our interview guide to the narrative flow of the conversation [34]. Thus, no two interviews were the same, and we continued to adapt and refine our thinking to reflect emerging themes from our ongoing analysis. As our research spanned the period of the COVID-19 pandemic, we actively considered how this affected our participants engagement with the project for P2 and P3, how community health interventions and national and international media campaigns may have shaped their understandings of health, hygiene and disease.

We took a purposeful and pragmatic approach to sampling and worked closely with our fieldwork assistants to identify men and women aged 18 years or over living in Kware, who were willing to talk to us about everyday health and hygiene [35]. Drawing on the principles of thematic saturation to determine final sample size we interviewed women from 11 households for P1. After our analysis of the P1 interviews, we resumed fieldwork in Kware for the two further phases, concluding that we had reached theoretical saturation after interviewing a further 42 people: 20 people in P2 and 23 in P3 [36]. The 53 participants included 35 females and 18 males, aged between 18 and 83 (see **Table 1**). The number of women included in our study reflects the gendered nature of social and economic roles, as many men were away from their homes during the day either at work or looking for work. However as gendered roles mean that women are often regarded as responsible for family and household hygiene, we do not regard this as a limitation of our study. Following advice from our fieldwork assistants, in P1 all participants were offered a single gift of body and clothes cleaning products (soap, shampoo etc.) to the value of $10 USD, presented at the end of the interview. For the second two phases of fieldwork (2021–2022) we were advised to give grocery store vouchers to the equivalent of $10, so that participants could decide on their immediate household needs.

The inductive and discursive interviews lasted between 30 minutes to over 1 hour and were audio-recorded with our participant's permission [34]. We followed the principles of informed consent, and after explaining the project to them in their language of choice we gave participants the opportunity to ask questions and then decline or accept our invitation to take part. Our research drew on theories of situated field ethics that focus on building trust and reducing inequalities between researchers and participants. We were responsive to our field assistant's guidance and our own judgments about the conduct of the research, and this shaped our approach to participants, the duration of the interviews and the direction of questioning etc. [37]. Our fieldwork included ethnographically informed observations of participant's homes and immediate surrounding areas, and these were recorded as fieldnotes [38]. We also gained consent to take photographs of home settings, household objects and spaces used for hygiene practices to gain a deeper understanding of resources and practices [39].

All interviews were later transcribed in the original languages (Kiswahili and English) and those in Kiswahili were also translated into English. All interview

Phases	Females	Males	Age range (years)
P1	11	—	18–58
P2	16	4	18–74
P3	8	14	18–83
Total	35	18	

Table 1.
Overview of participants.

transcripts were aurally checked and amended in English/ Kiswahili by Olivia Howland and Hamilton Majiwa. We imported the transcripts (English translations) into the qualitative data management tool NVivo (n = 53) to assist our analysis and to enable us to digitally share our ideas about the data [40]. Drawing on theories of inductive analysis, we created initial free codes by considering the content of each transcript word by word, and line by line. Jude Robinson and Hamilton Majiwa led the coding process with additional comments and suggestions from Olivia Howland. The agreed free codes were first refined, and then combined and merged to create theoretical and analytical themes [41]. We continues to discuss ideas, our coding and the nature of the themes throughout the three phases of data collection and analysis, considering any negative cases of alternative ideas, to reach a shared interpretation of our data [42].

2.2 Findings

Using the two intersecting themes of water security and water hygiene practices, we explore participants' knowledge and concerns, and the strategies they developed to mitigate the risks to their health. Ours is a qualitative research project and so while our interpretative themes represent the views of our participants, they are not generalizable to wider populations. Yet our depth approach enabled us to gain a sense of the range of strategies that people living in the same community have developed to mitigate the perceived hazards. Despite often living near one another, our participants responded to the same challenges in different ways, depending on the time, knowledge and physical and economic resources available to them at any point. It was evident that these responses were also seasonal, and that the local environment shaped water location and water hygiene practices. In the longer quotations of exchanges within interviews we present below, 'R' stands for respondent, and 'I' designates the interviewer.

As the research took place at three different time points, in December 2019, September 2021 and March 2022, we explicitly addressed how the ongoing COVID-19 pandemic may have altered hygiene behaviors and knowledge of disease. We did find evidence that behaviors had changed, particularly in the earlier stages of the pandemic in 2020, as more information and importantly, more resources were provided to the community. People described more frequent handwashing at the new handwashing stations and soap provided for residents, wearing masks and social distancing. By September 2021, much of the temporary infrastructure had been withdrawn from public places, and many participants said that they had resumed their former behaviors, and that nothing had changed. However increased knowledge of the importance of regular handwashing was mentioned by many participants and some described that they washed their hands more frequently than before the pandemic period:

> *Nothing has changed in fact the routine of hand washing has become more. Kw001 P2.*

> *Though for me I used to wash hands always in my household. But it has forced many people to take precaution and wash hands for sure. Kw002 P2.*

We found that in Kware, in common with many households worldwide, the sourcing and transportation of water and related household hygiene and health activities, such as washing, cooking and cleaning are largely performed by women, although we did find evidence that some men routinely helped with household chores.

As this participant recognizes, water is used for 'everything' for health and hygiene, including the preparation of many foods:

One only needs water since it is used for everything. That is why they say water is life. If we have water its fine since it is used for everything. If you don't have water you cannot even cook. We need water for everything. Kw004 P3.

This participant describes the many times she uses water in a single day, with calls on her time to clean the communal washing and latrine area, to washing the bodies and clothes of infants sometime multiple times each day, and to spend time boiling water to avoid serious illness for her children:

You know the bathroom has to be clean. So you might clean but someone else won't. You get it? Things like utensils can't stay dirty neither can't the kid especially when he urinates on himself. I don't know how he got it but after complaining about stomach upsets, he was diagnosed with typhoid and it was because of the water, so since then, I normally boil it. For instance, if this kid goes out there for a minute, he'll come back with a cold or even chest problems because of the wind. For instance, this one has to be washed daily or whenever he messes on himself but the older ones take a bath at least ones a day. Kw018 P1.

2.2.1 Water insecurity

Water insecurity was identified as a persistent problem for residents of Kware during all three phases of the research, reflected in discussions about the price of water, water quality and difficulties they experienced as they tried to access enough water for their daily household needs.

Sometimes one may not have money therefore lack water or at times you may have money and there is no water. Kw010 P3.

Sometimes there is water shortage. Like yesterday there was no water then today it came and we fetched but then we are forced to ration use of water. We are at times not able to take a full bath for lack of it. Kw016 P2.

There was clearly a hierarchy of water for many people, and they associated different water sources with different levels of risk and employed different storage and cleaning practices for their water depending on whether it was to be used for drinking, cooking or washing. While some knowledge of the levels of the relative risks was shared between households, practices varied according to income as some women simply could not afford the more desirable alternatives:

R: When it rains, we don't have to go fetch water. There is a drum where it drains into,

That is the water I use for all purposes

I: Is this water good for drinking?

R: We have no choice but to drink the water. When there's water one must bathe and drink. Kw003 P1.

Many participants described how they lacked the money to buy water at times and had to ration its use. Washing and bathing became less frequent, but at times, families were unable to afford to buy drinking water and relied on local sources for drinking. While everyone we spoke to knew of the need to boil water before drinking, the response from this participant suggests that local water sources were not always boiled:

> *If you do not have money to buy drinking water, you know there is water sold specifically for drinking. If you cannot afford, you just drink this one. When the child gets sick, you have to boil the water and give it while hot so as to kill the germs. It is not easy because I have to use kerosene or charcoal and it's expensive to buy. I use it sparingly Kw002 P1.*

Water pricing varied between sites and with the seasons and participants discussed the different options open to them on a daily basis, giving accounts of the many strategies that they developed to access water:

> *We go looking for it as far as the next road when there is none, there we are forced to buy drinking water only. Then we look for the donkey cart vendors to buy one for cooking, that means you have drinking water and that for cooking. Washing clothes, we go and borrow from the neighbour's borehole. Kw018 P3.*

Buying water from the itinerant vendors had the advantage that the water was brought to your door. This avoided the time and physical strength needed to make multiple trips to source water for intensive activities such as washing and was used by older or disabled people who could not carry the water themselves and did not have family close by. However this represents a more expensive option for them:

> *When there is no water there, I have a rough time because I cannot go looking for water. I ask a young man to go and buy some from the neighbours for me at 5/= then I pay him 10/= for every jerrycan he brings. Kw014 P3.*

> *Sometimes there is no water so we buy from donkey cart vendors who sell at between thirty shillings to forty shillings. Kw009 P3.*

Others described how in times of severe water and economic insecurity they would source local water from rivers and streams. They said that they would try to source from areas that looked cleaner, and would filter the water through cloth to let the sediment settle, but often were unable to boil the water and/or add purification tablets as they lacked money to access these resources:

> *I: Have you heard of people suffering from stomach problems after consuming water?*

> *R: Yes. It even happened in my house. We took them to hospital and it was because of water. The river water is not good. We only use it for washing clothes. Kw012 P2.*

2.2.2 Water hygiene practices:

Participants were concerned about water quality, but practices of water hygiene and perceptions of what constituted 'clean water' differed between households. The majority separated water for drinking from water for used for cooking, and some even differentiated between water for cooking and the water they used for different cleaning tasks. Water for drinking was often stored in a distinctive colored or marked container, usually made of plastic, and was often stored away from other water storage containers to further mark the distinction:

> *As of now we collect rainwater, but when there is no rain, we get water from the junction. The rainwater is used for laundry or cleaning the house. We buy drinking water and for cooking we get from the junction. This is like a ghetto; you cannot just drink any water... It is a specific blue bottle with a neck meant for storing drinking water. I store it here in the kitchen. Kw007 P1.*

Many people sourced their drinking water separately to their cooking and washing water and would pay a higher price for what was termed 'mineral water'. While a few participants claimed to buy drinking water in plastic bottles, the majority took their own drinking water containers to a trusted vendor where they would pay to have it refilled:

> *R: We have separate ones for drinking water, cooking water and water for washing clothes.*
>
> *I: Do you get the water from the same place for all these?*
>
> *R: No. drinking water we have a container which we refill with mineral water, for cooking we store in its drum then for washing clothes we store outside in another drum... Mineral water is treated but the one from the borehole you are not sure if it is treated. You are not sure if it has been put any chemicals down there. For mineral water one is sure the water went through the right procedure and is safe for use. Kw001 P2.*

Many of these strategies were time-consuming for the women and as water had to be carried, labour-intensive as well if water needed to be transported over longer distances. Often people settled for the closest source of water, even if there were concerns over water quality:

> *I: Is it the same water you use for cleaning, drinking and washing?*
>
> *R: That is for drinking and cooking. Washing we have water over there. While we were digging the toilet we got water and that's what we use. Kw014 P2.*

Some participants, mostly women, talked about cleaning the containers for drinking water more regularly than other containers, sometimes using soap to do so. People who did not have sealable containers for their water and used buckets were aware of storage issues, and so used different buckets for different purposes and avoided letting their drinking water stand for too long. They described how green slime could form and discolor the water and they actively prevented this, particularly to the water containers that they had reserved for their drinking water. However other people took their drinking and cooking water from the same source as their washing water, but their hygiene practices differed:

> *R: Some [jerrycans] hold washing water, some hold cooking water while some hold drinking water.*
>
> *I: What peculiarity does the one holding drinking water have?*
>
> *R: I always clean it Kw006 P1.*

Others were less likely to clean their jerrycans and it could be longer than a month before they washed them, even though they will have been refilled many times during that period:

I: How often do you clean these water jerrycans?

R: I will not lie because at times I stay for long without washing them.

I: Would you say a week or two?

R: That or sometimes even after a month. Kw016 P2.

Others did not source their drinking/cooking water separately from the water they used for cooking and cleaning, but stored it in a distinctive container, suggesting that they more actively monitored the quality of this water more than that stored in the other containers:

I: Why is it important to separate these jerricans?

R: To differentiate drinking water from the other water. I put drinking water in this drum then the rest is set aside for washing and other chores.

I: Do you treat the drinking water once stored in the drum?

R: No I just store it as it is. Kw015 P2.

Even though this water was identified as water for drinking, separation in terms of storage seems to be the only distinguishing factor and it was not treated in terms of boiling or the use of water purification tablets to improve it for consumption. As home water treatment requires both time and resource, the response from this participant suggests that they do not have additional money to source the water that they would ideally like to have in their home:

I: Do you boil water for drinking?

R. I feel it is safe to drink so I don't boil it.

I: Are you pleased with the quality of water you use?

R. Not as such. I feel it is safe because I can't afford the alternative but as the only option I choose to trust that it is safe for consumption. Kw008 P3.

Similarly, this participant did not use water from a different source, and did not keep a particular container for their drinking water:

I: When you are going to buy water, do you separate your jerricans, for example, a specific one for cooking and drinking?

R: No, the water is clean. Kw014 P2.

The majority of participants were mistrustful about water quality and referred to water from some sources not being 'clean' or being full of what they believed to be harmful 'chemicals'. Some of the water they bought that was piped from boreholes to sites in their community (tap water) was only used for bathing and cleaning:

R: We buy drinking water and the rest is used communally for chores.

I: Why is it important for you to buy drinking water?

R: This tap water is not trustworthy because at times it is not clean. Kw012 P2.

Some participants also complained that the water quality varied, and they were constantly sourcing and resourcing a water supply that they trusted to be clean:

R: Sometimes I do not always refill. At times this other water tastes too much chlorine. I decide at times because this refilled water is better quality and well treated to prevent diseases.

I: Are you worried that the other water may be contaminated?

R: Yes. I just do not trust it completely. Kw006 P3.

Most of our participants were aware that boiling water and/or treating water with water purification tablets made it suitable for drinking:

You cannot really say that this water is clean because you cannot really know its source. I don't normally use it for drinking and if I do, then I'll have to boil it Kw018 P1.

With a child you do not just give any water anyhow. Say if the vendor brings water and you do not know the source and the child has to drink it, I boil.... but fuel is a challenge... I am not confident because it sometimes causes sickness. We do not use it because we like to but only because we need to for lack of options. Kw012 P3.

Some had good supplies of water treatment tablets, often obtained from community health centers or the hospital if they had recently been there for treatment. Concerns about the quality of water and observations of the possibilities of contamination made people aware of the hazards of even piped water in their communities:

May be the precautions... is to ensure that kids don't get out of the gate because of the water... because if they go out and play they will obviously run in that water and it will be dangerous to them. So just making sure that they do not get out the gate is one of the precautions as well. And even the water that we drink we make sure that maybe we can put in Water Guard because you know... we buy water from a water tap, and the same water that we buy from there may be the same water running on the road... because of breakage of the pipes or something... so we make sure that the water is clean either by boiling or by putting Water Guard in the water just to ensure that we are safe. Kw005 P1.

2.3 Barriers and opportunities to improve water security and hygiene practices

Access to water is a challenge in this community. Most households do not have piped water and they buy water from water kiosks or water vendors who supply the water on donkey carts when the water kiosks have no water. During our research period in 2019–2022, water was sold for between 5 Kenyan Shillings (KSH), equivalent to USD 0.05, and KSH 20 (USD 0.20) for a 20 liters Jerrycan. This challenge of accessing water and the cost involved may lead to challenges in achieving the desired standards of hygiene as indicated by the responses of our participants.

Essentially, local ecologies shape everyday hygiene practices in households as people respond to diurnal and seasonal changes in their external environment. Living in areas of socio-economic disadvantage presents daily challenges to keeping clean. Periods of drought and/or flooding not only disrupt family hygiene practices but often contribute to a loss of income for the household, which means that families cannot afford the basic resources they need to keep themselves and others clean [43]. These accounts from multiple households of differing practices to secure water hygiene resonates with other research, which also found inequalities of water access even within informal settlements [44]. Inequalities of water access exist even within informal settlements [44], with those owning boreholes or those with relatively higher incomes having much better access to water (and potentially safer water) than those on lower incomes. Some participants reported using Water Guard, a liquid or tablet water treatment, yet for many, other needs took priority and they did not purify the water before drinking.

The issue of water quality was a concern for the study participants, and most did not trust the quality of the water. They used it only because they had no other options, due to access and/or financial constraints. Some participants boiled their water for drinking and added purification tablets to the water before using it to improve the quality, but others did not routinely do this. Participants had a good understanding of the risks involved in drinking untreated or un-boiled water but had little alternative due to constraints on their time, the cost of fuel, and/or their families disliking the taste. The risks of water borne diseases, such as typhoid, giardia and cholera, are reduced by strategies that improve the sourcing, storage and treatment of drinking water in areas of environmental disadvantage [45]. Participants recognized these risks but sometimes had to reduce washing of bodies, clothes and surfaces to conserve limited water supplies [46]. The COVID 19 pandemic led to increased water consumption [47] due to more regular hand washing practices and the need to wash surfaces regularly to avoid transmission. Yet in places like Kware, basic needs are prioritized over messages from global health advisories and recommendations may be disregarded by communities who cannot wash their hands or clean surfaces as often as they would like.

These complex issues of access to, and quality of, water are considered daily by women and men on lower incomes in Kware as they attempt to keep themselves, their families and their homes clean and healthy. Yet there is space within this narrative and context for opportunities to improve water security, health and hygiene. As we have demonstrated there is a good level of understanding of water and health, and the risks of using water from untrusted sources, but the primary issue is a lack of financial ability to access clean and safe drinking water. The organization of jerrycans for drinking, cooking and cleaning by some households is one positive way in which participants are actively prioritizing health within the constraints of their resources. Encouraging the boiling of water for drinking would further improve health as this is relatively inexpensive when compared to water treatment tablets or liquid (although time consuming when domestic chores are many). Improving access through reliable borehole supplies would also improve health and wellbeing. Much of the issue of access to clean and safe water needs to be addressed from a structural perspective, with governments providing the much-needed infrastructure, as individuals and communities are constrained by finances and equipment and so cannot provide solutions on the scale required.

As climate change increases pressure on water resources for humans, particularly in urban settings, the need to improve the quality of existing resources will increase, as will the need to explore and identify new sources of safe water for human consumption. This is a global issue but by shedding light on local realities of water and hygiene, like those in Kware, we are better able to understand the challenges faced by communities and individual households on a daily basis in order to inform the essential interventions which are required to maintain the health and wellbeing of communities worldwide.

Acknowledgements

We would like to sincerely thank the people of Kware who gave up their time to talk to us, and the contribution of our fieldwork assistants, Abdia Guyo Arero and Martha Nyambura. We would also like to thank the Sub-Chief's Office in Kware for their active and engaged support for our study. We would like to acknowledge the advice and contribution of our co-researchers, Ann Munene, Danait Solomon, Dr Annie Cook and Professor Nicola Williams to the Everyday Clean project. Thanks too for the support from the HORN project onehealthhorn.net at the University of Liverpool and the International Livestock Research Institute (ILRI), Kenya, particularly the help of Mark Lutton, Nik Cooper and Vicky Kyallo. This work was supported by the UK Research and Innovation, BBSRC Global Challenges Research Fund, Grant number **BB/P029954/1.**

Author details

Jude Robinson[1]*, Hamilton Majiwa[2] and Olivia Howland[3]

1 University of Glasgow, Glasgow, UK

2 University of Nairobi, Nairobi, Kenya

3 University of Liverpool, Liverpool, UK

*Address all correspondence to: jude.robinson@glasgow.ac.uk

References

[1] Bukachi SA et al. Exploring water access in rural Kenya: Narratives of social capital, gender inequalities and household water security in Kitui county. Water International. 2021;**46**(5):677-696

[2] United Nations. Sustainable Development Goals: Decade of Action. 2020. Available from: https://www.un.org/sustainabledevelopment/decade-of-action/. [Accessed: September 3 2020]

[3] Wutich A. Water insecurity: An agenda for research and call to action for human biology. American Journal of Human Biology. 2020;**32**(1):e23345

[4] Jury WA, Vaux HJ. The emerging global water crisis: Managing scarcity and conflict between water users, Advances in Agronomy. 2007;**95**:1-76

[5] Abram NJ et al. Connections of climate change and variability to large and extreme forest fires in Southeast Australia. Communications Earth & Environment. 2021;**2**(1):8

[6] Wu Y et al. Sand and dust storms in Asia: A call for global cooperation on climate change. The Lancet Planetary Health. 2021;**5**(6):e329-e330

[7] Eekhout JPC, de Vente J. Global impact of climate change on soil erosion and potential for adaptation through soil conservation. Earth-Science Reviews. 2022;**226**:103921

[8] Mukeka JM et al. Human-wildlife conflicts and their correlates in Narok County, Kenya. Global Ecology and Conservation. 2019;**18**:22

[9] Tabari H. Climate change impact on flood and extreme precipitation increases with water availability. Scientific Reports. 2020;**10**(1):13768

[10] Surasinghe T. The effects of climate change on global wildlife and terrestrial ecosystems. TAPROBANICA: The Journal of Asian Biodiversity. April 2010;**2**(1): 30-47

[11] Neumann JE et al. Climate effects on US infrastructure: The economics of adaptation for rail, roads, and coastal development. Climatic Change. 2021;**167**(3):44

[12] Ray DK et al. Climate change has likely already affected global food production. PLoS One. 2019;**14**(5):e0217148

[13] Kamta FN, Schilling J, Scheffran J. Water resources, forced migration and tensions with host communities in the Nigerian part of the Lake Chad Basin. Resources. 2021;**10**(4):27

[14] Kummu M et al. The world's road to water scarcity: Shortage and stress in the 20th century and pathways towards sustainability. Scientific Reports. 2016;**6**(1):38495

[15] Savelli E et al. Don't blame the rain: Social power and the 2015-2017 drought in Cape Town. Journal of Hydrology. 2021;**594**:125953

[16] Meehan K et al. Exposing the myths of household water insecurity in the global north: A critical review. WIREs Water. 2020;7(6):e1486

[17] Deitz S, Meehan K. Plumbing poverty: Mapping hot spots of racial and geographic inequality in U.S. household water insecurity. Annals of the American Association of Geographers. 2019;**109**(4):1092-1109

[18] UNA-UK. World Water Day—Factsheet. 2016. Available from:

https://una.org.uk/world-water-day-factsheet. [Accessed July 8 2022].

[19] Deshpande A et al. Mapping geographical inequalities in access to drinking water and sanitation facilities in low-income and middle-income countries, 2000-17. The Lancet Global Health. 2020;**8**(9):e1162-e1185

[20] van Vliet MTH et al. Global water scarcity including surface water quality and expansions of clean water technologies. Environmental Research Letters. 2021;**16**(2):024020

[21] Chua PLC et al. Associations between ambient temperature and enteric infections by pathogen: A systematic review and meta-analysis. The Lancet Planetary Health. 2022;**6**(3):e202-e218

[22] Charnley GEC, Kelman I, Murray KA. Drought-related cholera outbreaks in Africa and the implications for climate change: A narrative review. Pathogens and Global Health. 2022;**116**(1):3-12

[23] Pouramin P, Nagabhatla N, Miletto M. A systematic review of water and gender interlinkages: Assessing the intersection with health. Frontiers in Water. 2020;**2**:1-25

[24] Collins SM et al. 'I know how stressful it is to lack water!' Exploring the lived experiences of household water insecurity among pregnant and postpartum women in western Kenya. Global Public Health. 2019;**14**(5):649-662

[25] Drysdale RE, Bob U, Moshabela M. Coping through a drought: The association between child nutritional status and household food insecurity in the district of iLembe, South Africa. Public Health Nutrition. 2020;**24**(5):1052-1065

[26] Hayes K et al. Climate change and mental health: Risks, impacts and priority actions. International Journal of Mental Health Systems. 2018;**12**(1):28

[27] Cooper S et al. Environmental associated emotional distress and the dangers of climate change for pastoralist mental health. Global Environmental Change. 2019;**59**:101994

[28] Archambault CS. Women left behind? Migration, spousal separation, and the autonomy of rural women in Ugweno, Tanzania. Signs. 2010;**35**(4):919-942

[29] Démurger S. Migration and families left behind. IZA World of Labor. 2015:144. DOI: 10.15185/izawol.144

[30] Hasan SI et al. Prevalence of common mental health issues among migrant workers: A systematic review and meta-analysis. PLoS One. 2021;**16**(12):e0260221

[31] Campbell C. Migrancy, masculine identities and AIDS: The psychosocial context of HIV transmission on the South African gold mines. Social Science & Medicine. 1997;**45**(2):273-281

[32] Robinson J et al. The 'good life', personal appearance, and mental health of Congolese refugees in Rwanda and Uganda. Social Science & Medicine. 2021;**293**:114641

[33] Pols J. Washing the citizen: Washing, cleanliness and citizenship in mental health care. Culture, Medicine and Psychiatry. 2006;**30**(1):77-104

[34] Vindrola-Padrez C. Rapid Ethnographies. Cambridge: Cambridge University Press; 2020

[35] Vasileiou K et al. Characterising and justifying sample size sufficiency in interview-based studies: Systematic analysis of qualitative health research over a 15-year period. BMC Medical Research Methodology. 2018;**18**(1):148

[36] Baker S, Edwards R. How Many Qualitative Interviews is Enough?: Expert

Voices and Early Career Reflections on Sampling and Cases in Qualitative Research. 2012. National Centre for Research Methods Review Paper. Available from: http://eprints.ncrm.ac.uk/2273/4/how_many_interviews.pdf

[37] Perez TS. In support of situated ethics: Ways of building trust with stigmatised 'waste pickers' in Cape Town. Qualitative Research. 2019;**19**(2):148-163

[38] Emerson R, Fretz R, Shaw L. In: Atkinson P et al., editors. Participant Observation and Fieldnotes, in Handbook of Ethnography. London: Sage; 2007

[39] Pink S. Doing Visual Ethnography. London: Sage; 2007

[40] Bazely P. Qualitative Data Analysis: Practical Strategies. London: Sage; 2013

[41] Silverman D. Interpreting Qualitative Data. Thousand Oaks: Sage; 2012

[42] Pope C, Ziebland S, Mays N. Qualitative research in health care. Analysing qualitative data. BMJ. 2000;**320**(7227):114-116

[43] Bisung E, Elliott SJ. Improvement in access to safe water, household water insecurity, and time savings: A cross-sectional retrospective study in Kenya. Social Science & Medicine. 2018;**200**:1-8

[44] Oskam MJ et al. Socio-economic inequalities in access to drinking water among inhabitants of informal settlements in South Africa. International Journal of Environmental Research and Public Health. 2021;**18**(19):1-19

[45] McGuinness SL et al. Household water storage management, hygiene practices, and associated drinking water quality in rural India. Environmental Science & Technology. 2020;**54**(8):4963-4973

[46] Rieckmann A et al. Exploring droughts and floods and their association with cholera outbreaks in sub-Saharan Africa: A register-based ecological study from 1990 to 2010. American Journal of Tropical Medicine and Hygiene. 2018;**98**(5):1269-1274

[47] Staddon C et al. Water insecurity compounds the global coronavirus crisis. Water International. 2020;**45**(5):416-422

Chapter 2

Perspective Chapter: Access to Rural Water and Sanitation Services in Cameroon within the Context of Sustainable Development Goals (SDGs)

Victor Dang Mvongo, Paul Blaise Mabou, Célestin Defo, Paul Fabrice Nguema, Anil Kumar Mishra and Auguste Ombolo

Abstract

This chapter examines the situation of rural water and sanitation services in Cameroon within the context of sustainable development goals (SDGs), to establish whether Cameroon is on right track of meeting the SDG, and proposes actions to be taken to achieve universal access for water and sanitation. Based on the analyzed data obtained from national surveys and the Joint Monitoring Program for 2021, it argues that Cameroon is unlikely to reach universal access to water and sanitation in rural area by 2030. Factors contributing to poor access to rural water and sanitation services include the poor application of the policy and legal framework, the poor coordination of interventions between the actors involved in the sector, the low financial viability of the sector, the low efficiency of expenditure related to water and sanitation, and the lack of human resources in the sector. The implementation of the policy and legal framework, the stability of the institutional framework, the reaffirmation of the major role of the State of the changed Ministry of water, and the collaboration of all the actors of the sector within the mechanisms provided for this purpose are of fundamental importance to achieve SDG 6.1 and 6.2 in Cameroon.

Keywords: sustainability, water and sanitation governance, policy, rural development

1. Introduction

The recent report of the Joint Monitoring Programme for Water Supply, Sanitation and Hygiene (JMP) states that 771 million people in 2020 remain without access to basic water services and an estimated 1.69 billion without access to basic sanitation services [1]. The majority of people who still lacked even basic services lived in rural areas. Failure by governments to ensure access to basic water and sanitation services in rural areas is the result of a failure to ensure that infrastructure, once in place, continues to effectively provide the expected services over time [2]. For illustration, some studies [3, 4] have shown that 30–50% of rural water supply systems become inoperable 5 years after their construction.

The issue of the sustainability of rural water and sanitation services in Sub-Saharan Africa is not new and has received international attention since the International Decade of Potable Water and Sanitation (1981–1990). In this context, the focus to address rural water supply and sanitation systems failure was at the level of the community during the implementation phase of new facilities [2]. Since the Millennium Development Goals (MDG) era, emphasis has been placed on post-construction support to service providers, professionalization, and diversification of service delivery models [5].

With the adoption of the sustainable development goals (SDGs), governments have committed to ensure universal and equitable access to water and sanitation for all by 2030; to reduce inequalities in access to drinking water and sanitation; and to provide high levels of water and sanitation service in terms of quality, accessibility, and reliability. The SDGs thus pose a triple challenge, *viz.*, i) improving the levels of service provided; ii) ensuring the sustainability of services and promoting universal access to drinking water; and iii) sanitation [6]. In this context, it has become essential to better understand the factors of sustainability for rural water and sanitation services. Therefore, this chapter examine the situation of rural water and sanitation services in Cameroon within the context of sustainable development goals (SDGs), establish whether Cameroon is on track of meeting the SDG, identify factors that affect access to rural water and sanitation services, and proposes actions to be taken to achieve universal access for water and sanitation.

2. Country context

Cameroon is located in Sub-Saharan Africa between West and Central Africa at the extreme North Eastern end of the Gulf of Guinea (**Figure 1**). It lies between latitudes 2° and 13° North of the equator and between longitude 8° and 16° East of the Greenwich Meridian. It has a total surface area of 475,650 km^2 with a mainland surface area of 466,050 km^2 and a maritime surface area of 9600 km^2, respectively [7]. The estimated population is 27 million [1]. The rural population represent 41.3% of the total population. About 35% of the urban population lives in the economic capital, Douala, or the administrative capital, Yaoundé [8]. Administratively, Cameroon is divided into 10 regions, 58 divisions, and 360 sub-divisions. Cameroon has 14 cities and 360 councils.

Average GDP growth in real terms in Cameroon is around 4% over the past 5 years [9]. This development has not been sufficient to promote poverty reduction. Indeed, the population living below the poverty line is estimated at around 40%, which means that nearly half of the population is unable to access basic social services, including water [10]. This socioeconomic snapshot of the country has a direct impact on the Drinking Water, Hygiene and Sanitation sector. Indeed, the rate of access to drinking water is 66% while that of sanitation is 45% [1].

In rural areas, domestic water is supplied through wells and boreholes equipped with hand pumps and by rural distribution networks. Since 2010, the municipalities have been project owners and operators of facilities that are not part of the perimeter granted to the Cameroon Water Utilities Corporation (Camwater). However, the facilities remain in the domain of the State. Few data are available on the failures of

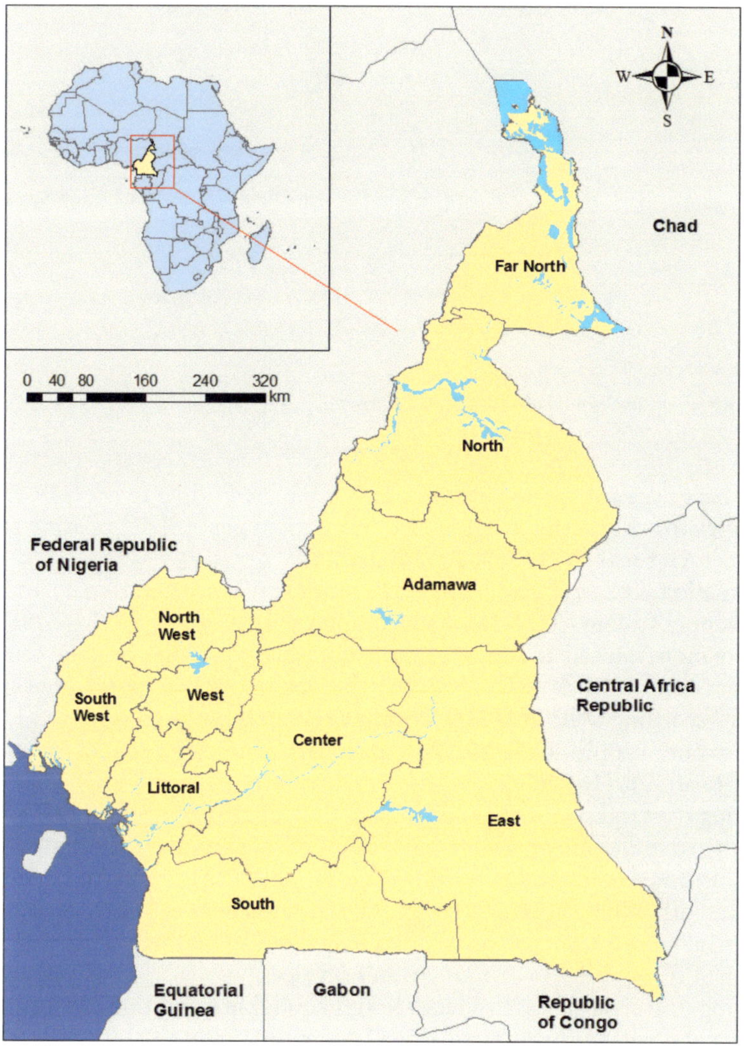

Figure 1.
Location of Cameroon.

rural water and sanitation system (RWSS). With the regard to sanitation, individual facilities including traditional latrines (receiving excreta, sewage and gray water) and improved facilities (ventilated single or double pit latrines and flush toilets connected to a septic tank) are the main sanitation facilities in rural areas.

3. Snapshot of the current state in terms of water and sanitation

In rural areas, very few data are available on access to drinking water and sanitation. The analysis presented in this section is based on data published by the Joint Monitoring Program (JMP) of WHO and UNICEF in 2021. According to these estimates, the rate of access to drinking water in rural has increased from 36.8% in 2000 to 43.5% in 2020, an increase of 6.7 points. About 6 million people living in rural areas

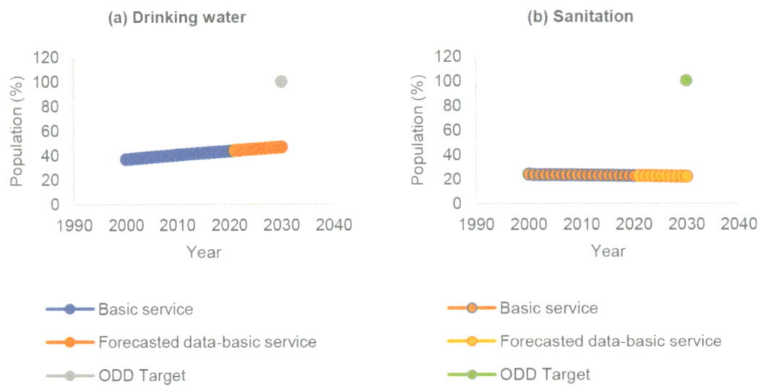

Figure 2.
Progress in water supply and sanitation coverage in Cameroon.

would not have access to an improved water source. According to the JMP, Cameroon is not on track to achieve the sustainable development goal (SDG) relating to drinking water (SDG 6.1), set at 100% in 2030 (**Figure 2a**).

This situation is exacerbated by the high number of non-functional rural drinking water supply system (RDWSS). Deal and Furey [11] estimated that 32% of hand pumps were inoperable at all times. In addition, isolated studies in some Cameroonian councils showed that 10–60% RDWSS were broken or not functioning optimally [6, 12–14]. According to RESEN [15], a third of schools in the country have a source of drinking water supply, while MINEDUB statistics indicate a school drinking water coverage rate of 39% [16] only.

Achieving the target 6.1 means addressing the **"unfinished business"** of extending services to 6 million people who still lack even a basic water service. It also implies going beyond households and providing access to services in schools, health-care facilities, and other institutional settings. The commitment to **"leave no one behind"** will require increased attention on disadvantaged groups and efforts to monitor elimination of inequalities in drinking water services.

Achieving universal access to adequate and equitable sanitation and hygiene by 2030 is a major challenge in rural areas in Cameroon. Target SDG 6.2 calls to end open defecation, to ensure that everyone has access to a basic toilet and to put in place systems for safe management of excreta. Based on an average population of 4.4 inhabitants per household and 1.8 households per plot served by a latrine, there would be approximately 330,197 improved facilities in rural areas. The sludge, in the absence of a fecal sludge treatment station, is discharged into the natural environment or, once the pit is full, it is sealed and a new pit is built near the previous one. The facilities of many public establishments (hospitals, schools, markets, etc.) are deficient.

Due to the rapid growth of the rural population, the rate of access to sanitation fell from 24.1% to 22.7% between 2000 and 2020, that is, a decline of 1.4 points. The country is therefore, to achieve the 100% fixed sanitation SDG seems to be difficult task (**Figure 2b**). The situation of poor access to water and sanitation services is accentuated by the many humanitarian crises affecting the country, i) internal and cross-border population displacements (Nigeria to Cameroon, Central African Republic to Cameroon), ii) nutritional and environmental crises (floods since 2012), iii) climate change and variability, and iv) health (cholera, polio, measles).

The health situation in the country has naturally been affected by the decline in access to sanitation facility. Thus, from 2009 to 2011, Cameroon experienced a serious epidemic of cholera, a fecal peril disease, and a second epidemic occurred in 2014. From 2009 to 2015, the country brought a total of 37,539 cases of cholera and 1694 deaths [17]. WHO estimates that diarrheal diseases due to poor drinking water supply, basic sanitation and hygiene practices cause 18,300 deaths per year and 13.4% morbidity in Cameroon [17].

4. Enabling and accelerating progress

This section focuses on the enablers for progress in the water and sanitation sector in rural areas in Cameroon and the challenges and obstacles faced, based on the MoI for water and sanitation (governance, finance, capacity development, data acquisition, and monitoring). They are interlinked and essential elements in meeting SDG targets for water and sanitation.

4.1 Policy and legal frameworks

4.1.1 Current status

Cameroon has many policy and strategy instruments, including the National Drinking Water Supply and Sanitation Policy in rural areas [18], the National Liquid Sanitation Strategy [19], and the National Community-Led Total Sanitation Strategy [17]. As for the legislative and regulatory framework, it is mainly based on Law No. 64/LF/23 of November 13, 64 on the protection of public health, Law No. 98/005 of April 14, 1998 on the water regime in the Cameroon, Law No. 2019/024 of December 24, 2019 on the general code of local authorities, and Decree No. 2010/0239/PM of February 26, 2010 setting the terms for the exercise of certain powers transferred by the State to the Municipalities in drinking water supply in areas not covered by the public water distribution network granted by the State.

The politico-legal framework analysis of the management of water and sanitation services in rural areas highlights many constraints and challenges. First of all, the obsolescence of the legal framework, in particular Law No. 64/LF/23 of November 13, 64 on the protection of public health and Law No. 98/005 of April 14, 1998 on the water regime. Indeed, with the changes in the socioeconomic and institutional landscape that Cameroon has experienced over the past two decades, these laws are proving obsolete. These laws are an extension of colonial legislation through which water and sanitation management follows Western models with a centralized management system [20]. In addition, there are discrepancies and even contradictions between the various texts governing water management in rural areas [17–19].

In addition to the question of the harmonization of laws and regulations governing the sector of management of rural water services in Cameroon, there is the problem of their applicability due to the fact either of the absence of implementing texts (decrees and decrees) or their pure and simple non-application despite the existence of laws and regulations [21]. Indeed, Law No. 98/005 of April 14, 1998 on the water regime in Cameroon provides for application decrees that are not all taken, and others not applied. This renders the application of this law obsolete. For illustration, the National Water Committee created by decree No. 2001/161/PM of May 8, 2001 and which is not fully functional, because it met only once, whereas the statutory provisions impose at least two regular meetings per year. The same is true for Law No. 2019/024 of December 24, 2019 on the general code of local authorities where there are not yet many implementing decrees such as the decree setting the procedures for exercising powers transferred by the State to the Communes in terms of sanitation in rural areas. Moreover, in the absence of sufficient financial resources, the national policy for drinking water supply and sanitation in rural areas has not, however, initiated any significant reform of the sector.

In addition, the context of the formalization of economic and social life, the weakness of the State's own means, makes it even more difficult to apply this normative system [22]. Moreover, the current legislative and regulatory texts do not mention the administration of water and sanitation in Cameroon [18]. The sector is still poorly "equipped" at the regulatory level. There is a lack of legislative and regulatory texts concerning the management of water and sanitation services. In addition, the place of rural sanitation in policy documents is very limited.

4.1.2 Accelerating progress

The analysis of the legal and institutional framework for the management of water and sanitation services shows that the legal basis for water and sanitation remains inconsistent and relatively inefficient. This legal basis is deemed insufficient and requires clarification, particularly with regard to the programming, construction, and ownership of the works. Significant efforts must be made to update and harmonize the political and legal framework for the management of water and sanitation services in rural areas. The ongoing review of Law N98/005 of April 14, 1998 on the water regime opens up prospects for taking into account the weaknesses identified and the establishment of a water and sanitation code. In addition, concerted efforts must be made to ensure greater effectiveness of the rich existing political and legal framework in the area of water and sanitation. Moreover, many efforts remain to be made to coordinate the implementation of various legislative and regulatory instruments in order to ensure synergy in this area, a source of efficiency in the interventions of the various actors.

4.2 Institutional arrangements

4.2.1 Current status

In Cameroon, the Ministry of Energy and Water (MINÉE) is responsible for the design, formulation and implementation of drinking water supply and sanitation strategies in rural areas. However, without a national policy or direction specifically dedicated to sanitation, the actions of the MINEE in rural areas are mainly oriented toward the construction of rural drinking water system and the organization of drinking water supply. In addition, the decentralized services of MINÉE experience difficulties in carrying out their mission (weak human and financial resources, difficulties in collaborating with local authorities, particularly in the area of WASH).

The main constraint of the institutional framework is the weak coordination of interventions between the MINÉE and the other Ministries involved in water and sanitation management and non-governmental organizations. Indeed, each of these actors intervenes with different logics and in quasi-autarky without coordination [17–19]; even if the National WASH Committee is in place, it struggles to assume the responsibilities of strong coordination of the sub-sector. Further, there is an overlap in the skills of MINEE in the management of water and sanitation services with other State structures. The lack of coordination between the public institutions of the State, having legal prerogatives of intervention in the field and the poor articulation between the functional levels, is sources of conflicts of competence, poor use of resources, and inefficiency [18].

Additionally, the centralized administrative organization and the unilateral "top-down" policy of the State also constitute to remain a major constraint. Indeed, the State has concentrated all the prerogatives in terms of water in the hands of these central or regional structures. Most of the water and sanitation programs piloted are in fact implemented centrally [18]. The drinking water supply and sanitation works are programmed on the basis of the available financial envelope and this programming is more guided by a concern for balance in the sharing of resources between the 10 regions of the country. State institutions in fact register requests from several sources: elites, deputies, or representatives of the populations. But the satisfaction of the needs expressed by the local actors is above all a function of their ability to influence decisions at the central level.

4.2.2 Accelerating progress

The stability of the institutional framework of the WASH sector, the reaffirmation of the major role of contracting authority under the State of the changed Ministry of water, and the collaboration of all the actors of the water sector and sanitation within the mechanisms provided for this purpose (the National Water Committee and the WASH sector group) are of fundamental importance to achieve SDG 6.1 and 6.2 in Cameroon. Thus, it is necessary to make the coordination mechanisms not only functional but also vibrant to provide for this purpose. The suggested interventions, in particular, are discussed below:

4.2.2.1 National Water Committee

The National Water Committee is an administrative body whose mission is to coordinate the actions of the main ministerial sectors involved in the water sector. It is made up of representatives of the main ministerial departments that play an important role in the field of water. It should play a pivotal role in the water sector under the new orientation of the institutional landscape which will let the ministerial departments formulate and implement their sectoral water strategies.

4.2.2.2 WASH Committee

The WASH Committee is responsible for providing multifaceted support to the administrations responsible respectively for water and public health, basic education, secondary education, and territorial administration. The WASH committee should be more proactive on the matters of concern to revamp the existing infrastructure and distribution networks so that the water supply and sanitation can play a strategic role in the fight against poverty. WASH Committee should aspire more to ensure advocacy with the Government, national and international institutions, and economic operators for support for the activities related to developing proper water supply, sanitation, and sewage treatment/disposal mechanism in the country.

4.2.2.3 Water information system unit

The Water Information System Unit is housed within the Water Resources Management Department, and it aggregates data from the Water and Sanitation sector in order to ensure reporting and tools decision support for investments in the sector. It is the focal point for monitoring SDG 6 in Cameroon. There is a need to develop and strengthen the data collection, analysis, and implementation of programs based on the correct felt needs of water supply and demand and this unit should reach to the aspirations for realizing the SD goals in water sector in the country.

4.3 Finance

Funding for water and sanitation in rural areas in Cameroon comes from three sources: i) tariffs, ii) taxes, and iii) transfers, known as the "three Ts." Tariffs typically come from user fees and household investments, covering self-supply solutions and household sanitation. Taxes are typically the largest source of funding in rural areas in Cameroon. "Taxes include all funding from public budgets allocated by governments (at the central or local levels) for investment, subsidies and general sector funding" [23]. Transfers involve financing from overseas in the form of official development finance (ODF), and contributions from NGOs and remittances [23].

4.3.1 Tariffs

Actually, cost recovery from tariffs is lower for water supply and almost absent for sanitation. Indeed, the financial flows generated by the sale of water are very low and do not cover most of the operation and maintenance costs. This situation contributes to the increase in the duration of repairs and to the increase in the rate of non-functionality of water supply infrastructures [24–26]. In addition, this situation is aggravated by an almost general absence of a culture of selling water. Indeed, the construction of a local water market depends on the willingness to pay of populations. However, this depends on several factors. First of all, the principle of payment for water appears in opposition to the shared values of peoples. Free water is associated with the representation that water is a gift from nature. Therefore, it is considered an inalienable resource that must be accessible to all. This conception is inseparable from the social dimension of water. In addition, the presence of other water points where access to water is free (traditional well, river, etc.) tends to have a negative impact on water demand from modern water points where access is chargeable [27].

[Note: In rural India, too the water is considered as nature's free gift but in urban areas where the piped water is being supplied it has become a chargeable commodity. The rates, however, are not substantial. Bottled water, however, is very costly but people who can afford to pay are willing to pay for assured quality of drinking water.

If the principle of payment for water is accepted in some localities in rural areas, there are difficulties related to its application. Indeed, social ties are strong and are linked to kinship and neighborhood relationships. It is difficult to refuse to provide water to a relative or neighbor who cannot afford it. In addition, for a long time, the State gave free water to the populations and it is now becoming very difficult to make users pay for the water service. This absence of the culture of the sale of water coupled with the ability of users to pay for the water service makes it possible to determine the willingness of the user to pay for water. Under such circumstances, while the water supply and sanitation network is being developed by the government exchequer without much return in monetary terms, we may think of positive impacts and indirect benefits such as the people will contribute more efficiently in nation building and overall GDP will move in positive direction if they remain healthy and do not fall sick as in case of non-existent of such facilities and services.

4.3.2 Taxes and transfers

The planning, budgeting, and execution of financing allocated to the water and sanitation sector have undergone significant variations over the years. Thus, for the improvement of access to drinking water, the Government and the technical and financial partners of the sector have been deploying for several years an investment effort in line with the achievement of the SDGs. This effort is estimated at 277.985 billion between 2007 and 2016, and 270.2 billion between 2007 and 2015 respectively for urban water supply, rural water supply, and sanitation [28]. The same is true for the liquid sanitation program, which requires an investment of around 285 billion FCFA (US $ 600 million) for the next 10 years.

However, the situation is worrying with regard to budgetary allocations. Indeed, in its public expenditure review conducted in April 2009, the World Bank noted for the drinking water supply and rural sanitation sector: "Neither *the Caisse Autonome d'Amortissement* (CAA), nor financial services, nor the technical services were able to provide data on allocations and executions of external resources, year by year for the period 2002–2007" [29].

In addition, the effectiveness of expenditure remains relatively poor: Control mechanisms are incomplete or inoperative, unit prices are higher than in comparable countries, the market is not attractive enough (due to administrative red tape and the corruption), and the number of structures built is relatively low: an average of around 700 water point equivalents [29]. The current low efficiency of spending means not only that there is a certain level of wastage of financing but also that the achievement of SDGs 6.1 and 6.2 is unrealistic.

Faced with this situation that could be detrimental to the achievement of SDG-6, the Government of Cameroon has initiated, with the support of UNICEF, a traceability survey of public expenditure in the water, hygiene, and sanitation sector. This initiative currently will not only improve the efficiency, impact, and equity of public action but also to advocate for an increase in the resources allocated by the government to the drinking water sector, the hygiene, and sanitation. In addition, as part of the UNICEF Government of Cameroon Cooperation Program for the period 2018–2020, the country will have a strategy for mobilizing the resources needed to finance the drinking water, hygiene, and sanitation sector. However, the implementation of this strategy is not yet perceptible.

4.4 Capacity development

With Cameroon joining the "Structural Adjustment Program" of the 1990s, the recruitment of executives for the benefit of the water and sanitation sector was frozen. This situation has resulted in a drastic reduction in the staff of the water and sanitation sector, jeopardizing the capacity of the public water administration to properly carry out its missions. The current situation reveals that the staff is insufficient in juxtaposition with the existing institutional framework and the missions assigned to the water and sanitation sector.

Furthermore, human resources are almost non-existent in the decentralized territorial communities. The vast majority of local authorities do not yet have qualified personnel able to assume the new missions assigned to them under decentralization [30]. In addition, the populations have weak participatory capacities. Illiteracy, lack of information, education, and communication among rural populations are main obstacles to their conscious and responsible participation in the sustainable management of infrastructure and even water resources. The private sector exists in the construction of structures, but the quality of the structures built by them is often deficient due to the lack of normative documents, quality control, and experienced personnel [31].

In view of the above, it is important that the capacities of all actors involved in the management of water services in rural areas be strengthened. In this perspective, it is worth mentioning the establishments of initial, continuous, or professional training in the water and sanitation professions, which can be mobilized in particular the State Universities and the Private Institutes of Higher Education (IPES), the Training Center for Municipal Actors (CEFAM), strengthens the technical capacities of municipal staff and the National Training Program for City Trades (PNFMV). In addition, recruitment of additional staff and sensitization of users should be undertaken. Raising user awareness will enable water users to take an active part in the water service management process.

4.5 Data acquisition and monitoring

4.5.1 Current status

Cameroon through the Ministry of Economy, Planning and Regional Development (MINEPAT), with the support of the United Nations System, led in 2015, the process of inclusive localization of the SDGs. At the end of this process, the development actors gave their opinion on the relevant targets for Cameroon based on two main criteria, which are anchoring in development strategies and policies and taking into account the challenges emerging. As a logical follow-up to this, the National SDG-6 indicator framework for Cameroon was developed in October 2018. It presents the measurement indicators for each target, the data sources, the actors in charge of data collection, the analysis, and dissemination of indicators. However, the data currently available on access to drinking water supply, hygiene, and sanitation (WASH) services are those from surveys conducted as part of the JMP and MICS (Multiple Indicator Cluster Survey). These surveys are done by sampling and often do not reflect reality. Also, the estimates are not disaggregated according to the guidelines of the SDG implementation monitoring system.

To take into account the particularity and the complexity of the calculation of the SDG-6 indicators and more particularly indicators 6.1 on access to drinking water and 6.2 on basic sanitation, Cameroon has a WASH Infrastructure Data Management System housed in the Water Information System Unit and initiated in 2015 the inventory and geolocation of infrastructure. The information relates to the type, location, functionality, and management method of the structures and will ultimately be used to calculate the indicators to measure the level of achievement of SDG-6. However, the results of this inventory initiated with the help of the African Development Bank are not yet available and the mechanism for monitoring SDG-6 at the national level is not yet operational.

4.5.2 Accelerating progress

"We cannot plan and manage what we do not measure and monitor" is a statement that few would disagree with. Data acquisition and monitoring provide the foundation for good governance [23]. It is not possible to plan, manage, and evaluate rural water and sanitation services without available data. Cameroon lack the financial, institutional, and human resources to acquire and analyze data to support governance. The mechanism put in place to monitor the implementation of SDG-6 is not yet operational. Efforts must therefore be made to make this mechanism operational. In addition, on the basis of the main guidelines of the Monitoring and Accountability Supervision Framework, it is necessary to finalize the development of the framework for monitoring simplified indicators of progress toward SDG-6 by the populations themselves. In addition, annual sector reviews should be held with all the technical and financial partners involved in the management of water and sanitation services in rural areas. This could be done, for example, within the framework of the WASH cluster.

5. Conclusion

This chapter provides information on access to rural water and sanitation services in Cameroon. Analysis of data from the MICS surveys and the JMP 2021 suggests that at the current rate, it will be highly difficult to achieve SDG 6.1 and 6.2 in rural areas of Cameroon. Data analysis also suggests that factors such as i) weak application of the politico-legal framework for the management of water and sanitation services, ii) weak coordination of interventions between actors involved in the sector, iii) weak financial viability of the management of water and sanitation services, iv) the low efficiency of expenditure related to water and sanitation, and the v) insufficiency of human resources in the sector constitute major barriers to the achievement of the universal access to water and sanitation in rural areas.

Further, strengthening the implementation of the politico-legal framework, upgradation and modernizing the stability of the institutional framework of the WASH sector, ensuring the reaffirmation of the major role of Project Owner under the State of the changed Ministry of Water, and the whole hearted concerted efforts to ensure the collaboration of all actors/players in the water and sanitation sector within the mechanisms provided for this purpose (The National Water Committee and the WASH sector group) are of fundamental importance to achieve SDG 6.1 and 6.2 in Cameroon. While achieving a surmounting task is difficult yet not impossible, the need of hour is to start the much required action to achieve targets. We are quite optimistic and convinced that with the help and support of people of Cameroon and guidance of experts within or outside the country and finances generated from within the country or external support, achieving SDG-6 can be a reality 1 day provided most honest and sincere efforts are made till the goal is achieved.

Conflict of interest

The authors declare no conflicts of interest.

Acronyms and abbreviations

AMCOW	African Ministerial Council on water
CAA	*Caisse Autonome d'Amortissement*
GDP	Gross Domestic Product
JMP	Joint Monitoring Programme for water supply, sanitation and Hygiene

MICS	Multiple Indicator Cluster Survey
MINEDUB	Ministry of Basic Education
MINÉE	Ministry of Energy and Water
RWSN	Rural Water Supply Network
RWSS	Rural Water and Sanitation System
SDG	Sustainable development goals
UNICEF	United Nation International Children Emergency Fund
WASH	Water, Sanitation and Hygiene
WHO	World Health Organisation

Author details

Victor Dang Mvongo[1*], Paul Blaise Mabou[2], Célestin Defo[3], Paul Fabrice Nguema[3], Anil Kumar Mishra[4] and Auguste Ombolo[3]

1 Faculty of Agronomy and Agricultural Sciences, Department of Agricultural Engineering, University of Dschang, Dschang, Cameroon

2 Department of Geography, University of Dschang, Cameroon

3 Advanced School of Agriculture, Forestry, Water Resources and Environment, University of Ebolowa, Ebolowa, Cameroon

4 Water Technology Centre, Indian Agricultural Research Institute, New Delhi, India

*Address all correspondence to: victordangmvongo@gmail.com

References

[1] WHO, UNICEF. Progress on Household Drinking Water, Sanitation and Hygiene 2000-2020: Five Years into the SDGs. Joint Monitoring Program. Geneva, Switzerland: WHO Publishing; 2021

[2] World Bank. Sustainability Assessment of Rural Water Service Delivery Models: Findings of a Multi-Country Review. Washington, DC: World Bank; 2017

[3] RWSN. Myths of the Rural Water Supply Sector. Perspectives Paper No. 4, RWSN Executive Steering Committee. RWSN: St Gallen; 2010

[4] Improve International. Statistics on Water and Sanitation System Failures. 2012. Available from: http://improveinternational.wordpress.com/handy-resources/sad-stats

[5] Lockwood H, Smits S. Supporting Rural Water Supply: Moving towards a Service Delivery Approach. Rugby: Practical Action Publishing; 2011

[6] Mvongo VD, Defo C. Assessing water service performance in rural sub-Saharan Africa environment: The cases studies of two councils of the southern and eastern regions of the Republic of Cameroon (Central Africa). Journal of Water Sanitation and Hygiene for Development. 2021;**11**(1):37-50

[7] NIS (National Institute of Statistics). Cameroon Statistical Yearbook 2000. Yaoundé′-Cameroon: Ministry of the Economy and Finance; 2001

[8] Ako AA, Shimada J, Eyong GET, Fantong YW. Access to potable water and sanitation in Cameroon within the context of millennium development goals (MDGS). Water Science & Technology. 2010;**61**(5):1317-1339

[9] NIS (National Institute of Statistics). Enquête par grappes à indicateurs multiples (MICS5), 2014, Rapport Final. Yaoundé, Cameroun: Institut National de la Statistique; 2015

[10] NIS (National Institute of Statistics). Quatrième Enquête Camerounaise auprès des Ménages: ECAM 4. Yaoundé, Cameroun: Institut National de la Statistique; 2014

[11] Deal PT, Furey SG. RWSN International Directory of Rural Water Supply Models, Tariffs and Lifecycle Costs. 2019th ed. Skat Foundation, St. Gallen: RWSN; 2019

[12] Mvongo VD, Fonkou T, Defo C. Sustainability of water and sanitation services in Mandjou's council, East-Cameroon. In: 6th International Conference on Science & Technology of PKFokam Institute of Excellence, 11-June 2019, Yaoundé Cameroon. 2019

[13] Minlo FR, Defo C. Assessing the performance and strategy improvement of the water distribution network of the urban environment of Ebolowa, Cameroon. In: 5th International Conference on Science & Technology of PKFokam Institute of Excellence, 12-14 June 2018, Yaoundé Cameroon. 2018

[14] Tedah D, Defo C. Sustainable community water supply in rural area in Cameroon: A novel strategy for potable water point maintenance. In: 5th International Conference on Science & Technology of PKFokam Institute of Excellence, 12-14 June 2018, Yaoundé Cameroon. 2018

[15] RESEN. Le système d'éducation et de formation du Cameroun dans la perspective de l'émergence. 2013

[16] MINEDUB (Ministry of Basic Education). Education de Base en Chiffre. Edition 2013-2014. 2014

[17] MINEE (Ministry of Energy and Water). Stratégie nationale de l'assainissement total piloté par la communauté. 2017

[18] MINEE (Ministry of Energy and Water). Politique nationale d'approvisionnement en eau potable et assainissement en milieu rural. 2009

[19] MINEE (Ministry of Energy and Water). Stratégie d'assainissement liquide. 2011

[20] Fonjong LN. 2008. Gender roles and practices in natural resource management in the north West Province of Cameroon. Local Environment. 2008;**13**(5):461-475

[21] Kouam GR, Hernanie GM, Samuel AN, Serges LDB, Georges EE. Gestion Intégrée des Ressources en Eau et Objectives du Millénaire Pour le Développement en Afrique: cas du Cameroun. VertigO-La revue des sciences de l'environnement. 2006;7(2):1-9

[22] MINEE (Ministry of Energy and Water). Politique nationale de l'eau: rapport diagnostique du secteur de l'eau. 2017

[23] United Nations. Sustainable Development Goal 6 Synthesis Report 2018 on Water and Sanitation. New York; 2018

[24] Mvongo DV, Defo C, Tchoffo M. Application of water service sustainability index to water services in sub-Saharan Africa: The cases studies of eight councils in southern region of Cameroon (Central Africa). Journal of Water, Sanitation and Hygiene for Development. 2022;**12**(2):168-185. DOI: 10.2166/washdev.2022.157

[25] Foster T. Predictors of sustainability for community-managed handpump in sub-Saharan Africa: Evidence from Liberia, Sierra Leone, and Uganda. Environmental Science and Technology. 2013;**47**:12037-12046

[26] Harvey P. 2007 cost determination and sustainable financing for rural water services in sub-Saharan Africa. Water Policy. 2007;**9**(4):373

[27] Mvongo VD, Fonkou T, Defo C. Etude des modes d'approvisionnement en eau potable et stratégies de rehabilitation des points d'eau modernes ruraux en zone tropicale humide: cas de la Commune de Mvangan au Cameroun. VertigO-La revue des sciences de l'environnement. 2022;**22**(2):1-19. Available from: http://journals.openedition.org/vertigo/36164. DOI: 10.4000/vertigo.36164

[28] MINEE. Plan d'action 2008-2015 pour le secteur d'approvisionnement en eau potable et d'assainissement. 2008

[29] AMCOW (African Ministerial Council on Water). Approvisionnement en eau potable et assainissement au Cameroun: traduire les financements en services à l'horizon 2015 et au-delà. 2011

[30] MINEE, GWP-Cmr. Etat des lieux du secteur de l'eau au Cameroun: cadre financier, économique et social (tome 3). Yaoundé, Cameroun; 2009

[31] MINEE, GWP-Cmr. Etat des lieux du secteur de l'eau au Cameroun: cadre légal et institutionnel (tome 4). Yaoundé, Cameroun; 2009

Chapter 3

Typhoid in Less Developed Countries: A Major Public Health Concern

Tigist Gashaw and Abera Jambo

Abstract

Typhoid fever remains a major public health concern in less developed countries. The disease is transmitted through the consumption of food or water contaminated with feces containing Salmonella Typhi. *Salmonella* is a genus of the family *Enterobacteriaceae* with over 2450 species. Typhoid is more common in impoverished areas with unsafe drinking water sources and poor sanitation. These problems are further exacerbated by political instabilities, displacement, and war in the regions. Each year, 17.8 million cases of typhoid fever are reported in lower-income countries. Typhoid was expected to be most common in western Africa, followed by a few countries in Central, South, and Southeast Asia. In most cases, the incidence peaked between the ages of under 5 years. Recently, many *Salmonella* species had developed resistance to several antibiotics which call for serious prevention and control efforts that integrate several high-impact interventions targeting facilities and infrastructure, together with parallel efforts directed at effective strategies for use of typhoid conjugate vaccines. Hence, a multisector collaboration and approach from a different perspective have to be advocated for the containment of typhoid. The clinical and public health concerns and the strategies to stem the growing flows associated with typhoid are going to be discussed.

Keywords: typhoid, developing countries, antimicrobial resistance, typhoid conjugate vaccine, sanitation, hygiene

1. Introduction

Typhoid fever is an infection of the gastrointestinal tract, particularly the intestinal lumen, and it may involve the bloodstream [1]. Typhoid and paratyphoid fever are caused by gram-negative bacteria known as Salmonella typhi and *Salmonella Paratyphoid*, respectively, with the latter causing less severe disease, and they pose serious health problems to humans [2–4]. Eating contaminated food or drinking contaminated water is the main pathway through which these bacteria can spread [5, 6]. Typhoid fever is among the most common foodborne diseases and remains the major health problem in low-income countries while become declined in developed countries because of improved sanitation, safe food, and water [7–10].

1.1 Epidemiology of typhoid fever

Even if there is a drastic decrease in typhoid fever-related morbidity and mortality with improved living conditions and the introduction of antibiotics, the disease continues to be a public health problem in areas of Africa, the Americas, Southeast Asia, and the Western Pacific regions [11–13]. It is predicted that about 17.8 million cases of typhoid fever occur each year in low- and middle-income countries with Central Africa predicted to experience the highest incidence followed by Central, South, and Southeast Asia [14, 15].

It was also estimated that 14·3 million cases of typhoid and paratyphoid fevers occurred globally in 2017. Comparing global burden diseases (GBDs) super-regions, south Asia had the highest age-standardized incidence rate followed by Southeast Asia, western sub-Saharan Africa, eastern sub-Saharan Africa, and Oceania. Besides, South Asia had the largest number of cases, accounting for 71·8% of global cases followed by Southeast Asia, western sub-Saharan Africa, eastern sub-Saharan Africa, and East Asia as depicted in table below. Considering age, incidence rates were highest among children, peaking in 5–9 year ages. With 12.6% of cases occurred among children younger than 5 years and 55.9% occurred among children younger than 15 years [16].

Furthermore, it was estimated that 135·9 thousand deaths from typhoid and paratyphoid fever globally in which 85.9% were attributable to *S. typhi* in 2017 (**Table 1**). South Asia had showed the highest mortality rate with highest absolute of deaths 69.6% followed by sub-Saharan Africa super-region 15.9%, South Asia, East Asia, and Oceania super-region 12.3% of global death. In addition, mortality rates were highest among young children, with 17.2% of deaths occurred in younger 5 years and 59.3% under 15 years old. Considering sex, 74.0 thousand deaths occurred among males compared with 61.9% thousand death among females [16].

1.2 Clinical presentation and diagnostic consideration of typhoid fever

The clinical presentations of typhoid fever vary with the age of the patients as well as whether complications are present or absent [17]. Initially, patients may present with fever which is gradual in type and rises to 39–40°C at the end of the first week of disease onset [18]. Patients with typhoid fever present with gastrointestinal (GI) symptoms like nausea and vomiting, constipation, diarrhea, and abdominal pain [19, 20]. Patients may also present with non-GI symptoms like headache, skin rash, cough, and malaise [4]. Fever is the only frequent sign seen among under 5 years children unless the patient is presented with complications [19]. Nonspecific physical findings like soft and tender hepatosplenomegaly, distended abdomen, ascites, and diffuse/localized tenderness may also be noticed upon physical examination. Hepatitis and hepatomegaly are more common among children aged under 5 years, whereas constipation is common among adults [18, 21]. Some rare clinical features like bradycardia which may be secondary to high persistent fever, rose spots, and blanching erythematous maculopapular lesions on the trunk were also reported among patients with typhoid fever [22–24]. In the diagnosis of typhoid fever, in addition to the presenting symptoms, a culture test is considered [25].

1.3 Complications of typhoid fever

A severe form of the disease manifests in the second/third week of the illness with persistent fever, anemia, weight loss, increasing weakness, and persistent

	Cases (thousands)	Incidence (per 100,000)	Death (typhoid fever)
Global	14,321 (12540–16,337)	197·8 (172·0–226·2)	85·9% (77·7–91·9)
Central Europe, Eastern Europe, and Central Asia			
Central Asia	0·1 (0·1–0·1)	0·1 (0·1–0·1)	48·9% (22·2–87·2)
Central Europe	1·2 (0·9–1·5)	0·7 (0·6–0·9)	62·6% (47·0–80·1)
Eastern Europe	1·1 (0·9–1·5)	0·4 (0·3–0·5)	41·8% (27·0–62·7)
High income			
Australasia	0·0 (0·0 to 0·1)	0·2 (0·1–0·2)	39·2% (14·0–58·2)
High-income Asia Pacific	0·7 (0·6 to 0·9)	0·3 (0·2–0·3)	34·1% (18·0–73·8)
High-income North America	4·1 (3·2 to 5·3)	0·9 (0·7–1·2)	18·6% (6·2–30·5)
Southern Latin America	0·5 (0·4 to 0·6)	0·7 (0·5–0·9)	97·7% (92·8–99·0)
Western Europe	1·3 (1·0 to 1·6)	0·3 (0·2–0·4)	84·3% (77·1–96·4)
Latin America and Caribbean			
Andean Latin America	0·9 (0·7–1·1)	1·5 (1·2–2·0)	98·8% (97·8–99·4)
Caribbean	2·5 (2·1–3·0)	5·7 (4·7–6·7)	56·3% (40·7–70·4)
Central Latin America	20·0 (16·6–24·6)	8·2 (6·9–10·2)	98·3% (94·3–99·6)
Tropical Latin America	4·3 (3·3–5·5)	1·9 (1·5–2·4)	98·7% (97·6–99·3)
North Africa and Middle East	246·6 (210·8–286·3)	39·3 (33·7–45·6)	98·4% (97·2–99·2)
South Asia	10,286 (9002–11,738)	549·2 (480·7–625·4)	83·4% (73·9–90·3)
Southeast Asia, East Asia, and Oceania			
East Asia	586·6 (553·8–624·0)	51·0 (47·3–55·1)	76·9% (65·3–86·0)
Oceania	20·5 (17·0–24·7)	144·3 (121·5–170·4)	87·2% (79·4–92·9)
Southeast Asia	1414·4 (1247·9 to 1592·9)	219·8 (192·9–249·1)	94·5% (90·4–97·0)
Sub-Saharan Africa			
Central sub-Saharan Africa	122·4 (100·2–149·1)	81·4 (68·8–95·8)	98·5% (97·4–99·2)
Eastern sub-Saharan Africa	739·5 (627·6–869·7)	151·9 (132·0–174·6)	99·1% (98·3–99·5
Southern sub-Saharan Africa	1·9 (1·7–2·1)	2·3 (2·0–2·6)	95·5% (92·3–97·6)
Western sub-Saharan Africa	866·1(719·7–1039·6)	161·1(138·1–187·3)	84·8% (76·2–91·4)

Table 1.
Global and regional numbers of cases, incidence and deaths by year 2017 for typhoid and paratyphoid fevers [16].

GI manifestations (vomiting) [18]. Unless treated early, typhoid fever may also lead to encephalopathy, nephritis, GI bleeding, and hepatitis [26–28]. So, early initiation of appropriate treatment helps to reduce the chance of developing such complications.

2. Factors associated with typhoid fever

Different factors were associated with typhoid fever including individual, environmental, and socioeconomic-related factors. Accordingly, individual-related factors like a decreased gastric acid barrier and taking medications that decrease gastric acidity and a history of *Helicobacter pylori* infection increase the chance of acquiring typhoid fever [10]. In addition to this, poor hygiene practices in an individual as well as in the community level increase the likelihood of acquiring the disease [29]. Among environmental factors, the risk of acquiring typhoid fever is associated with being exposed to solid waste disposal on the field, nearby open sewers and contaminated water bodies, being a resident of low elevation areas, and the rainy season [29–31]. Different socioeconomic factors also increase the risk of acquiring typhoid fever. Those being user of spring and river water, and use of pit latrine, as well as individuals with low income, were more likely to get infected [32–34].

3. Impacts of typhoid fever

Typhoid fever is the result of a human host-restricted *Salmonella* enteric serotype *Typhi* infection that causes enteric fever [35]. Antibiotics are commonly used to treat typhoid fever, and early initiation of effective antimicrobial therapy has been shown to reduce disease duration as well as the risk of complications and death [36]. Clinicians may prescribe antibiotics to patients who do not have a confirmed diagnosis, based on clinical suspicion, due to the high risk of morbidity and mortality if untreated [37]. Large surveillance studies from Asia and Africa, on the other hand, show that only 1–4% of people with suspected typhoid have culture-confirmed typhoid [38], implying that unnecessary antibiotics are commonly used. Empiric antibiotic treatment has been shown to increase selection pressure on *Salmonella Typhi* (*S. Typhi*) [39]. As a result, with rising rates of treatment failure, antibiotic resistance has emerged as a major threat to typhoid treatment [40–42].

Different researchers are witnessing the full-blown resistance development toward former first-line antimicrobials against typhoid fever [43–45]. A similar pattern of resistance is also increasing toward the fluoroquinolones (ciprofloxacin) accounting for up to 80% of isolates [43, 45, 46]. Moreover, the backups cephalosporin (ceftriaxone and cefotaxime) is also in question marking up to 50% resistance in some specific areas [41]. Fortunately, the susceptibility of Azithromycin has been retained in many areas [46]. Though the potency of Carbapenems is still present [46], there is emerging evidence of resistance to Morepenem in a few findings [41]. In some areas, patients were wrongly diagnosed and treated for enteric fever by the Widal test. Rapid tests with better sensitivity and specificity are needed for the diagnosis of enteric fever [44]. Consequently, the magnitude of multiple and extended drug resistances is increasing in developing countries [47].

Multidrug resistance (MDR) refers to resistance to first-line antibiotics chloramphenicol, co-trimoxazole (trimethoprim-sulfamethoxazole), and ampicillin. In *S. Typhi,* complex MDR elements can be found on self-transmissible plasmids encoding an antibiotic resistance gene cassette or incorporated into the chromosome [48, 49]. While antibiotic selection keeps resistance genes on plasmids, there appears to be competition between plasmids encoding the same resistance trait [50]. Because of the spread of the specific H58 lineage across Asian and African countries, MDR *S. Typhi* has become common in many low-income countries, particularly in South and Southeast Asia [51–53]. Antimicrobial susceptibility patterns, like illness incidence, also vary spatially [54].

4. Preventions

Typhoid fever is a preventable disease. However, it continues to affect many populations across the globe. The biggest illness burden is seen in regions with low socioeconomic development, limited access to clean water, sewage and water management systems, poor sanitation standards, and other social risk factors such as population displacement, armed conflict, and natural disasters [55]. Hence, public health and clinical measures, which include improvements in water quality and sanitation [35], the deployment of *S. Typhi* vaccination and an informed choice of treatment must be implemented [56]. Reporting antimicrobial susceptibility testing is also imperative to facilitate evidence-based policy and practice to avert drug-resistant [52].

4.1 Vaccine

There are several vaccines available for the prevention of typhoid, the choice of which will include factors such as the local availability and age of the intended recipient. The World Health Organization (WHO) recommends the programmatic use of typhoid vaccines for the control of typhoid fever [57]. The three typhoid vaccines now in use globally are the unconjugated polysaccharide vaccine (Vi-PS), and the older generation typhoid conjugate vaccine (TCV) containing the Vi-polysaccharide antigen, and vaccination based on the injection of oral live attenuated *Salmonella strain* Ty21a [58]. TCV is the preferred formulation at the moment due to its immunological properties, wider application (can be given to infants as young as 6 months), and longer-lasting protection after a single dose. The TCV formulation has addressed some of the issues that previously hampered the effectiveness of both polysaccharide and live vaccines [59]. To stimulate the immune system more strongly, the *S. Typhi* Vi-polysaccharide is coupled to a protein in this formulation.

The Vi-TT and Vi-CRM197 formulations are the first typhoid vaccines approved for use in children under the age of 2 years, and several TCVs have been licensed on a national scale [60]. They are WHO-approved for use in infants as young as 6 months old [61]. Because of the high number of young children who contract typhoid fever, this approval was significant. The WHO recommends giving TCVs to children as a single dose at 9 months of age or in their second year of life in typhoid fever-endemic countries [57, 62].

4.1.1 Challenges, opportunities, and ways forward

Because typhoid is endemic in low-income countries, the greatest demand for vaccines is expected to come from the public sector, where financial incentives for vaccine manufacturers are limited. It will be difficult to keep manufacturers interested in TCV production and even more difficult to generate interest in the development of newer generation vaccine candidates [63]. Vaccine introduction and programmatic cost for vaccination are other burdens. Besides, the lack of sufficient diagnosis as well as surveillance data on disease pathogenesis [64], drug susceptibility, and typhoid vaccine effectiveness further challenged these regions [65].

Fortunately, recent finding from clinical studies in Africa, Malawi, is starting to sparkle a light on TCV effectiveness [66]. Besides, Liberia becomes the first country in Africa to introduce TCV with a weeklong campaign to reach more than 1.9 million children aged 9 months to younger than 15 years old. After the campaign, the country determines to integrate TCV into the routine immunization program for all children at 9 months old [67].

Vaccinations must compete for funding within health ministry's alongside other health objectives because they typically provide a good return on investment. This is especially true if the total public health benefits of a vaccine have been calculated [68]. In the case of typhoid vaccines, this would include indirect protection of those who have not received the vaccine, a reduction in antibiotic use, and a reduction in the development of antibiotic-resistant organisms [69]. Moreover, limiting health inequities and the moral capital the vaccines generate, decreasing outbreaks and the health care delivery distortions, and minimizing economic consequences from the loss of business or tourism when an outbreak occurs are all factors that will reduce the risk of household poverty as a result of the cost of treating typhoid [55, 70].

4.2 Water, sanitation, and hygiene

Water, sanitation, and hygiene (WASH) are critical for human health. Despite this, over 884 million people worldwide lack access to safe drinking water. Almost 2.4 billion people do not have access to even the most basic sanitary facilities. Many people practice open defecation, endangering the safety of drinking water and personal water supplies. Babies and young children are more likely to die if they do not have access to safe drinking water. Many diarrheal illnesses are caused by contaminated water and poor sanitation. These conditions can lead to the deadly diseases typhoid fever and cholera. Poor WASH conditions are also linked to new issues such as drug-resistant typhoid fever [71, 72].

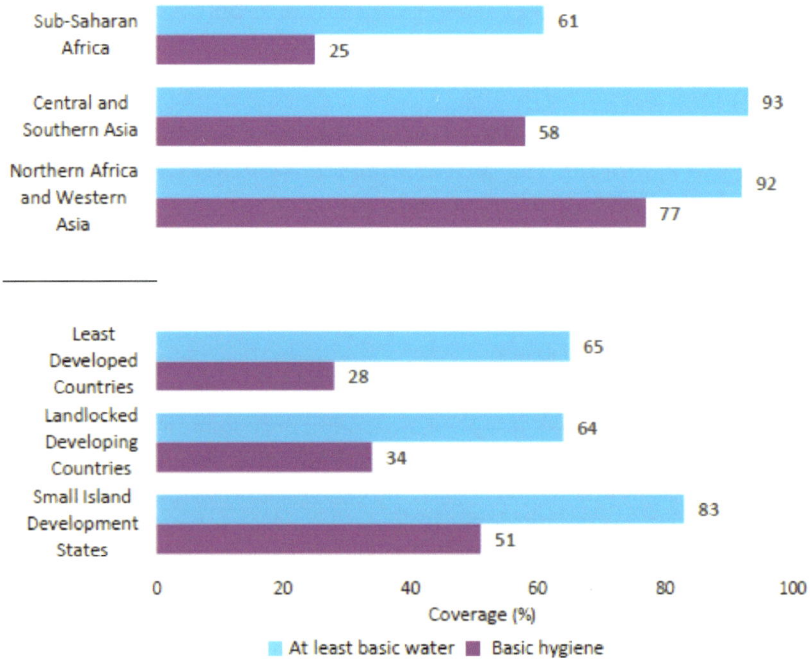

Figure 1.
Access to at least basic water services and hygiene services at home for regions with available national representative data, SDG regions, and other regional grouping 2017 [73].

Five years into the sustainable development goals (SDGs), the world is still on track to miss SDG target 6 (access to safe water and sanitation). To achieve universal coverage, current rates of advancement in properly managed drinking water services, securely managed sanitation services, and basic hygiene services must be quadrupled by 2030. Least-developed countries (LDCs) still have the most work to do, and accelerating progress in volatile environments will be especially difficult. Many more countries are struggling to provide services to their poor and vulnerable citizens, who are particularly at risk of being left behind (**Figure 1**) [73, 74].

Though international organizations and programs have been attempting to improve infrastructure as well as access to better sanitation and hygiene services focusing on schools [75, 76], it remained to be a key area of intervention [77] in reducing typhoid risk among children. Besides, insufficient funding and budgeting have been cited as major barriers to successfully integrating and maintaining WASH programs in school settings [78]. Involving the community by increasing user responsibility for program management and maintenance was one of the most crucial strategies to improve sustainability once funders or private financiers were no longer involved. By promoting community involvement, it may be simpler to make use of local resources, develop local WASH capacity, and guarantee user satisfaction [78, 79]. A significant reduction in typhoid risk has also been linked to the implementation of TCV programs and practical, culturally relevant family WASH practices [80].

5. Conclusions

A multidisciplinary strategy of public health based on personal protection and infrastructure interventions is needed. As typhoid vaccines do not offer complete protection, safe water, sanitation, and hygiene interventions are critical to preventing the spread of typhoid. Other efforts might be directed toward effective treatment options, to provide care as early as possible to achieve better outcomes. Additionally, as there is often limited awareness and knowledge of infectious diseases in affected populations, hence, education and community engagement should be considered.

Conflict of interest

The authors declare no conflict of interest.

Acronyms and abbreviations

S. Typhi	*Salmonella Typhi*
GBD	global burden diseases
MDR	multidrug resistance
GI	gastrointestinal
TCV	typhoid conjugate vaccine
WASH	water, sanitation, and hygiene
SDGs	sustainable development goals
WHO	World Health Organization

Author details

Tigist Gashaw[1*] and Abera Jambo[2]

1 Department of Pharmacology and Toxicology, School of Pharmacy, College of Health and Medical Sciences, Haramaya University, Harar, Ethiopia

2 Clinical Pharmacy Department, School of Pharmacy, College of Health and Medical Sciences, Haramaya University, Harar, Ethiopia

*Address all correspondence to: yekalabel@gmail.com

References

[1] Sheikh A, Charles RC, Sharmeen N, Rollins SM, Harris JB, Bhuiyan MS, et al. In vivo expression of salmonella enterica serotype Typhi genes in the blood of patients with typhoid fever in Bangladesh. PLoS Neglected Tropical Diseases. 2011;**5**(12):e1419

[2] Harris JB, Brooks WA. Typhoid and Paratyphoid (Enteric) Fever. Hunter's Tropical Medicine and Emerging Infectious Diseases. Amsterdam, Netherlands: Elsevier; 2020. pp. 608-616

[3] Kuijpers LM, Phe T, Veng CH, Lim K, Ieng S, Kham C, et al. The clinical and microbiological characteristics of enteric fever in Cambodia, 2008-2015. PLoS Neglected Tropical Diseases. 2017;**11**(9):e0005964

[4] Habte L, Tadesse E, Ferede G, Amsalu A. Typhoid fever: Clinical presentation and associated factors in febrile patients visiting Shashemene referral hospital, southern Ethiopia. BMC Research Notes. 2018;**11**(1):1-6

[5] Ligon BL, editor. Infectious diseases that pose specific challenges after natural disasters: A review. In: Seminars in Pediatric Infectious Diseases. Amsterdam, Netherlands: Elsevier; 2006

[6] Ashbolt NJ. Microbial contamination of drinking water and disease outcomes in developing regions. Toxicology. 2004;**198**(1-3):229-238

[7] Musoke D, Namata C, Lubega GB, Niyongabo F, Gonza J, Chidziwisano K, et al. The role of environmental health in preventing antimicrobial resistance in low- and middle-income countries. Environmental Health and Preventive Medicine. 2021;**26**(1):100

[8] Eng S-K, Pusparajah P, Ab Mutalib N-S, Ser H-L, Chan K-G, Lee L-H. Salmonella: A review on pathogenesis, epidemiology and antibiotic resistance. Frontiers in Life Science. 2015;**8**(3):284-293

[9] Faour-Klingbeil D, Todd CD, E. Prevention and control of foodborne diseases in middle-east north African countries: Review of national control systems. International Journal of Environmental Research and Public Health. 2020;**17**(1):70

[10] Manesh A, Meltzer E, Jin C, Britto C, Deodhar D, Radha S, et al. Typhoid and paratyphoid fever: A clinical seminar. Journal of Travel Medicine. 2021;**28**(3):taab012

[11] Kothari A, Pruthi A, Chugh TD. The burden of enteric fever. The Journal of Infection in Developing Countries. 2008;**2**(04):253-259

[12] Buckle GC, Walker CLF, Black RE. Typhoid fever and paratyphoid fever: Systematic review to estimate global morbidity and mortality for 2010. Journal of global health. 2012;**2**(1):-010401

[13] Otegbayo J. Typhoid fever: The challenges of medical management. Annals of Ibadan Postgraduate Medicine. 2005;**3**(1):52-54

[14] Carvalho MS, Antillón M, Warren JL, Crawford FW, Weinberger DM, Kürüm E, et al. The burden of typhoid fever in low- and middle-income countries: A meta-regression approach. PLOS Neglected Tropical Diseases. 2017;**11**(2):e0005376

[15] Collaborators GTaP. The global burden of typhoid and paratyphoid

fevers: A systematic analysis for the global burden of disease study 2017. The Lancet Infectious Diseases. 2019;**19**:369-381

[16] Stanaway JD, Reiner RC, Blacker BF, Goldberg EM, Khalil IA, Troeger CE, et al. The global burden of typhoid and paratyphoid fevers: A systematic analysis for the global burden of disease study 2017. The Lancet Infectious Diseases. 2019;**19**(4):369-381

[17] Connor BA, Schwartz E. Typhoid and paratyphoid fever in travellers. The Lancet infectious diseases. 2005;**5**(10):623-628

[18] Basnyat B, Qamar FN, Rupali P, Ahmed T, Parry CM. Enteric fever. BMJ. 2021;**372**:n437

[19] Basnyat B. Tackling typhoid fever burden in South Asia. The Lancet Global Health. 2022;**10**(7):e932-e9e3

[20] Jamil B, Lashari I, Bhatti S, Hasan RS. Enteric fever in adult patients: Clinical features, outcome and antibiotic susceptibility patterns. Infectious Disease Journal of Pakistan. 2004;**13**:68-72

[21] Balter S. Typhoid Fever, Acute and Carrier. Acute Communicable Disease Control 2016 Annual Morbidity Report. Los Angeles: CDC; 2016

[22] Lee B, Rose E. Other Potentially Life-Threatening Conditions with Mucocutaneous Findings (Leptospirosis, Typhoid Fever, Dengue, Diphtheria, Murine Typhus): Life-Threatening Rashes. Vol. 12. The Capital Region of Denmark: Springer, Cham; 2018. pp. 319-347. DOI: 10.1007/978-3-319-75623-3_23

[23] Kang JH. Febrile illness with skin rashes. Infection & Chemotherapy. 2015;**47**(3):155-166

[24] Lasheen RA, ElTohamy A, Salaheldin EO. MIS-C frenzy: The importance of considering a broad differential diagnosis. SAGE Open Medical Case Reports. 2022;**10**:1-5

[25] Wijedoru L, Mallett S, Parry CM. Rapid diagnostic tests for typhoid and paratyphoid (enteric) fever. Cochrane Database of Systematic Reviews. 2017;**5**:CD008892

[26] Pramoolsinsap C, Viranuvatti V. Salmonella hepatitis. Journal of Gastroenterology and Hepatology. 1998;**13**(7):745-750

[27] Anand AC, Garg HK. Approach to clinical syndrome of jaundice and encephalopathy in tropics. Journal of Clinical and Experimental Hepatology. 2015;**5**:S116-SS30

[28] Azmatullah A, Qamar FN, Thaver D, Zaidi AK, Bhutta ZA. Systematic review of the global epidemiology, clinical and laboratory profile of enteric fever. Journal of Global Health. 2015;**5**(2):020407

[29] Akwa TE, Nguimbous SP. Investigation of typhoid fever and their associated risk factors in children attending "Deo Gratias" Hospital in Douala, Littoral, Cameroon. European Journal of Medical and Educational Technologies. 2021;**14**(2):em2107

[30] Dewan AM, Corner R, Hashizume M, Ongee ET. Typhoid fever and its association with environmental factors in the Dhaka metropolitan area of Bangladesh: A spatial and time-series approach. PLoS Neglected Tropical Diseases. 2013;7(1):e1998

[31] Baker S, Holt KE, Clements AC, Karkey A, Arjyal A, Boni MF, et al. Combined high-resolution genotyping and geospatial analysis reveals modes of endemic urban typhoid fever transmission. Open Biology. 2011;**1**(2):110008

[32] Irda Sari SY, Sunjaya DK, Shimizu-Furusawa H, Watanabe C, Raksanagara AS. Water sources quality in urban slum settlement along the contaminated river basin in Indonesia: Application of quantitative microbial risk assessment. Journal of Environmental and Public Health. 2018;**2018**:3806537

[33] Hamner S, Tripathi A, Mishra RK, Bouskill N, Broadaway SC, Pyle BH, et al. The role of water use patterns and sewage pollution in incidence of water-borne/enteric diseases along the Ganges River in Varanasi, India. International Journal of Environmental Health Research. 2006;**16**(2):113-132

[34] Dungumaro EW. Socioeconomic differentials and availability of domestic water in South Africa. Physics and Chemistry of the Earth, Parts A/B/C. 2007;**32**(15-18):1141-1147

[35] Akram J, Khan AS, Khan HA, Gilani SA, Akram SJ, Ahmad FJ, et al. Extensively drug-resistant (XDR) typhoid: Evolution, prevention, and its management. BioMed Research International. 2020;**2020**:6432580

[36] Diniz-Santos DR, Silva LR, Silva N. Antibiotics for the empirical treatment of acute infectious diarrhea in children. Brazilian Journal of Infectious Diseases. 2006;**10**:217-227

[37] Veeraraghavan B, Pragasam AK, Bakthavatchalam YD, Ralph R. Typhoid fever: Issues in laboratory detection, treatment options & concerns in management in developing countries. Future science OA. 2018;**4**(6):FSO312

[38] Andrews JR, Baker S, Marks F, Alsan M, Garrett D, Gellin BG, et al. Typhoid conjugate vaccines: A new tool in the fight against antimicrobial resistance. The Lancet Infectious Diseases. 2019;**19**(1):e26-e30

[39] Tatavarthy A, Luna VA, Amuso PT. How multidrug resistance in typhoid fever affects treatment options. Annals of the New York Academy of Sciences. 2014;**1323**(1):76-90

[40] Crump JA, Sjölund-Karlsson M, Gordon MA, Parry CM. Epidemiology, clinical presentation, laboratory diagnosis, antimicrobial resistance, and antimicrobial management of invasive salmonella infections. Clinical microbiology reviews. 2015;**28**(4):901-937

[41] Shah SAA, Nadeem M, Syed SA, Abidi STF, Khan N, Bano N. Antimicrobial sensitivity pattern of salmonella Typhi: Emergence of resistant strains. Cureus. 2020;**12**(11):e11778

[42] Sartelli M, Weber DG, Ruppé E, Bassetti M, Wright BJ, Ansaloni L, et al. Antimicrobials: A global alliance for optimizing their rational use in intra-abdominal infections (AGORA). World journal of emergency surgery. 2016;**11**(1):1-32

[43] Mutai WC, Muigai AW, Waiyaki P, Kariuki S. Multi-drug resistant salmonella enterica serovar Typhi isolates with reduced susceptibility to ciprofloxacin in Kenya. BMC Microbiology. 2018;**18**(1):1-5

[44] Deksissa T, Gebremedhin EZ. A cross-sectional study of enteric fever among febrile patients at ambo hospital: Prevalence, risk factors, comparison of Widal test and stool culture and antimicrobials susceptibility pattern of isolates. BMC Infectious Diseases. 2019;**19**(1):1-12

[45] Mashe T, Gudza-Mugabe M, Tarupiwa A, Munemo E, Mtapuri-Zinyowera S, Smouse SL, et al. Laboratory characterisation of salmonella enterica serotype Typhi

isolates from Zimbabwe, 2009-2017. BMC Infectious Diseases. 2019;**19**(1):1-9

[46] Hughes MJ, Birhane MG, Dorough L, Reynolds JL, Caidi H, Tagg KA, et al. Extensively Drug-Resistant Typhoid Fever in the United States. Open Forum Infectious Diseases. US: Oxford University Press; 2021

[47] Butt MH, Saleem A, Javed SO, Ullah I, Rehman MU, Islam N, et al. Rising XDR-typhoid fever cases in Pakistan: Are we heading Back to the pre-antibiotic era? Frontiers in Public Health. 2022;**9**:794868

[48] Duy PT, Nguyen TNT, Thuy DV, Alcock F, Boinett C, Thanh HND, et al. Ciprofloxacin facilitates the transfer of XDR plasmids from commensal E. coli into epidemic fluoroquinolone-resistant Shigella sonnei. bioRxiv. 2019:767251 [Preprint]

[49] Sarwar Y, Ali A, Haque A, Haque A. Current status of antimicrobial resistance in enteric bacterial pathogens. Frontiers in Clinical Drug Research: Anti-Infectives. 2014;**1**:263

[50] Vogwill T, MacLean RC. The genetic basis of the fitness costs of antimicrobial resistance: A meta-analysis approach. Evolutionary Applications. 2015;**8**(3):284-295

[51] Azhar AB, Khalid A, Shah S. The implications of extensive drug-resistant typhoid fever: A case report. Cureus. 2019;**11**(6):e5032

[52] Browne AJ, Kashef Hamadani BH, Kumaran EA, Rao P, Longbottom J, Harriss E, et al. Drug-resistant enteric fever worldwide, 1990 to 2018: A systematic review and meta-analysis. BMC Medicine. 2020;**18**(1):1-22

[53] Masuet-Aumatell C, Atouguia J. Typhoid fever infection–antibiotic resistance and vaccination strategies: A narrative review. Travel Medicine and Infectious Disease. 2021;**40**:101946

[54] Frost I, Van Boeckel TP, Pires J, Craig J, Laxminarayan R. Global geographic trends in antimicrobial resistance: The role of international travel. Journal of Travel Medicine. 2019;**26**(8):taz036

[55] Khan MI, Franco-Paredes C, Sahastrabuddhe S, Ochiai RL, Mogasale V, Gessner BD. Barriers to typhoid fever vaccine access in endemic countries. Research and Reports in Tropical Medicine. 2017;**8**:37

[56] Parry CM, Ribeiro I, Walia K, Rupali P, Baker S, Basnyat B. Multidrug resistant enteric fever in South Asia: Unmet medical needs and opportunities. BMJ. 2019;**364**:k5322

[57] WHO. Typhoid vaccines: WHO position paper–march 2018. Weekly Epidemiological Record. 2018;**93**:477-500

[58] Emergent BioSolutions U. Vivotif-Summary of Product Characteristics (SmPC)-(Emc). London: Emergent BioSolutions UK; 2018

[59] Neuzil KM, Pollard AJ, Marfin AA. Introduction of typhoid conjugate vaccines in Africa and Asia. Clinical Infectious Diseases. 2019;**68**(Supplement_1):S27-S30

[60] Sahastrabuddhe S, Saluja T. Overview of the typhoid conjugate vaccine pipeline: Current status and future plans. Clinical Infectious Diseases. 2019;**68**(Supplement_1):S22-SS6

[61] Lau CL, Streeton CL, David MC, Sly PD, Mills DJ. The tolerability of a combined hepatitis a and typhoid vaccine in children aged 2-16 years: An observational study. Journal of Travel Medicine. 2016;**23**(2):tav023

[62] Bentsi-Enchill AD, Hombach J. Revised global typhoid vaccination policy. Clinical Infectious Diseases. 2019;**68**(Supplement_1):S31-SS3

[63] Syed KA, Saluja T, Cho H, Hsiao A, Shaikh H, Wartel TA, et al. Review on the recent advances on typhoid vaccine development and challenges ahead. Clinical Infectious Diseases. 2020;**71**(Supplement_2):S141-SS50

[64] Yang Y-A, Chong A, Song J. Why is eradicating typhoid fever so challenging: Implications for vaccine and therapeutic design. Vaccine. 2018;**6**(3):45

[65] Venkatesan P. A trial of a typhoid conjugate vaccine in children in Malawi. The Lancet Microbe. 2021;**2**(12):e654

[66] Patel PD, Patel P, Liang Y, Meiring JE, Misiri T, Mwakiseghile F, et al. Safety and efficacy of a typhoid conjugate vaccine in Malawian children. New England Journal of Medicine. 2021;**385**(12):1104-1115

[67] Birkhold M, Mwisongo A, Pollard AJ, Neuzil KM. Typhoid conjugate vaccine in Africa and Asia: Status of clinical evaluation and vaccine introduction. The Journal of Infectious Diseases. 2021;**224**:S781-S787

[68] Shakya M, Neuzil KM, Pollard AJ. Prospects of future typhoid and paratyphoid vaccines in endemic countries. The Journal of Infectious Diseases. 2021;**224**(Supplement_7):S770-S7S4

[69] Saha SK, Tabassum N, Saha S. Typhoid conjugate vaccine: An urgent tool to combat typhoid and tackle antimicrobial resistance. The Journal of Infectious Diseases. 2021;**224**(Supplement_7):S788-SS91

[70] Steele AD, Carey ME, Kumar S, MacLennan CA, Ma L-F, Diaz Z, et al. Typhoid conjugate vaccines and enteric fever control: Where to next? Clinical Infectious Diseases. 2020;**71**(Supplement_2):S185-SS90

[71] CDC. Assessing Access to Water & Sanitation. Obtenido de Centers for Disease Control and Prevention. USA: CDC; 2017

[72] Bangert M, Molyneux DH, Lindsay SW, Fitzpatrick C, Engels D. The cross-cutting contribution of the end of neglected tropical diseases to the sustainable development goals. Infectious Diseases of Poverty. 2017;**6**(1):1-20

[73] WHO. Progress on Household Drinking Water, Sanitation and Hygiene 2000-2020: Five Years into the SDGs. Geneva: WHO; 2021

[74] WHO. Progress on Household Drinking Water, Sanitation and Hygiene 2000-2017: Special Focus on Inequalities. New York: World Health Organization; 2019

[75] World Health Organization. Achieving Quality Universal Health Coverage through Better Water, Sanitation and Hygiene Services in Health Care Facilities. Geneva: WHO; 2017

[76] IRC U. Towards Effective Programming for WASH in Schools: A Manual on Scaling up Programmes for Water, Sanitation and Hygiene in Schools. Delft, The Netherlands: IRC International Water and Sanitation Centre; 2007

[77] Seid H, Kumie A. The status of school sanitation facilities in some selected primary and secondary schools in Dessie City Administration, south Wello zone, Amhara region. Ethiopian Journal of Health Development. 2013;**27**(1):80-84

[78] McGinnis SM, McKeon T, Desai R, Ejelonu A, Laskowski S, Murphy HM.

A systematic review: Costing and financing of water, sanitation, and hygiene (WASH) in schools. International journal of Environmental Research and Public Health. 2017;**14**(4):442

[79] Alexander KT, Zulaika G, Nyothach E, Oduor C, Mason L, Obor D, et al. Do water, sanitation and hygiene conditions in primary schools consistently support schoolgirls' menstrual needs? A longitudinal study in rural western Kenya. International Journal of Environmental Research and Public Health. 2018;**15**(8):1682

[80] Tadesse BT, Khanam F, Ahmed F, Im J, Islam M, Kim DR, et al. Prevention of typhoid by vi conjugate vaccine and achievable improvements in household WASH: Evidence from a cluster-randomized trial in Dhaka, Bangladesh. Clinical Infectious Diseases. 2022;**74**:ciac289

Chapter 4

Maintaining Hand Hygiene in the Informal Settlements: Reflections on Compliance for Covid-19 Preventative Measures

Fhumulani M. Mulaudzi, Nombulelo V. Sepeng, Ndivhaleni R. Lavhelani and Tintswalo V. Nesengani

Abstract

South Africa experiences challenges with informal settlements that have inadequate water supplies and sanitation measures, thus affecting people's health status. As countries globally aim to attain Sustainable Development Goals 3 and 6, it is necessary to recognise how human well-being is significantly dependent on safe drinking water, sanitation and hygiene. Poor sanitation and an inadequate water supply to areas where people live lead to poor hygiene that may cause illnesses like diarrhoea. In this chapter, we reflect on the challenges that we faced during the Covid-19 pandemic and the effects on the practice of good hygiene. We used information from grey literature such as newspapers, reports from districts and radio interviews to extract stories from community members who experienced constraints in maintaining hygienic conditions during Covid-19. Results revealed that constraints, such as being confined in a shack, a lack of running water and poor sanitation affected community members' compliance to Covid-19 preventive measures.

Keywords: Covid-19, informal settlement, preventative measures, sanitation, water, sanitation

1. Introduction

The Covid-19 pandemic reached South African shores in 2020. The country was placed in a state of disaster management. Control and preventive measures were put in place to control the spread of Covid-19. Movements were restricted, resulting in the total lockdown of the country which was later managed through stages. The communities were made aware that the Covid-19 infection was spread by inhalation of infected droplets and contact with infected surfaces [1]. Different methods, such as social distancing, handwashing, use of sanitisers to maintain aseptic techniques to prevent the spread of the infection were introduced. The centres for disease control and prevention recommended and emphasised handwashing with soap and water for 20 seconds, repeatedly throughout the day. Other methods, such as the use of alcohol-based hand sanitisers, were also recommended [2]. Hand hygiene has always been a method that has been used in hospitals and clinics to prevent infection. However, COVID-19 put the practice into the spotlight for hand washing to be practiced by each and every member of society. This practice became a challenge, especially for people who are staying in informal settlements where issues such as social distancing and availability of running water remains a challenge.

In 2018/2019 the World Health Organisation (WHO) led an initiative to collect data on how governments and external support agencies (ESAs) worldwide are supporting hygiene [3]. Data was collected by the UN-Water Global Analysis and Assessment of Sanitation and Drinking-Water (GLAAS) [4]. The results of this initiative revealed that countries worldwide have put national policies and plans in place for hygiene; however, there is a lack of infrastructure to supply water and proper sanitation in certain areas [4]. Also, the sustainable development goal number 6 reads "*ensure availability and sustainable management of water and sanitation for all by 2030*" [5]. Despite that, water remains a scarce commodity in sub-Saharan Africa. Nearly 300 million people live in a water-stressed environment. In some countries, such as Kenya, people had to queue to get water, making it difficult for them to use the rationed water to wash hands frequently under running water, as expected, instead of bathing and cooking [6].

In South Africa, the issue of water remains a challenge caused by "insufficient water infrastructure maintenance and investments, inequities in access to water and sanitation, deteriorating water quality, and a lack of skilled water engineers and scientists". The Covid 19 pandemic and the prescribed preventive measures showed the inequities in water supply and sanitation. The Department of Water and Sanitation provided approximately 41,000 water tanks to assist people living in informal settlements and rural communities to assist with running water during the Covid-19 era [7]. However, this practice is not sustainable when the country is no longer reporting high incidences of Covid-19.

The practice of handwashing with soap and water seems an easy and simple thing to do in countries that have running water. However, in developing countries, such as South Africa, where water is a scarce commodity, the practice is viewed as a luxury that is often impossible to attain. Water scarcity is a big challenge in the fight of the spread of Covid-19, especially for those people staying in the informal settlements. Water scarcity causes unhygienic conditions and poor sanitation that affects vulnerable people, like children, and encourages diseases, such as diarrhoea, cholera, malaria, and in this case, the spread of Covid-19 [8]. Health care professionals working in informal settlements are also unable to comply with the maintenance of aseptic techniques to curb the spread of infections. This issue of water scarcity does not align with the sustainable development goal number 3 that reads "*Ensure healthy lives and promote wellbeing for all at all ages*".

South Africa is one of the countries that became an epicentre for Covid-19. Maintaining a clean and healthy environment in a place where people live in overcrowded conditions, the lack of water and basic sanitation is a challenge to the control of infection. Most of the poor people in South Africa live in informal settlements, such as squatter camps, rondavels and shacks. People living in informal settlements get water from outside taps and the toilets are outside their houses and they are communal which made it more difficult for them to comply with the preventive measures that were in place to promote hand hygiene and the spread of the Covid-19 virus [8]. Developed countries, such as Australia, suspended water shut-offs and closure for water access for those who were in debt to ensure water access [9]. Other developing countries, such as Ghana, spent money on water tanks to provide water to their communities during Covid-19 to make water available for hand washing to prevent the spread of the virus [9].

The importance of ensuring access to safe Water, Sanitation and Hygiene (WASH) was viewed as a priority to prevent the spread of Covid-19 infection. In this chapter, we reflect on the challenges experienced by people living in informal settlements regarding compliance to Covid 19 preventive measures in South Africa.

2. Research design and methods

An integrated literature review was used to obtain information regarding this topic. The keywords used were Covid-19, informal settlement, preventative measures, hand sanitizers, water scarcity, Wash. The websites used were EbscoHost, google scholar, Pubmed and CINAHL. We accessed articles from 2019 to 2022. We found 83 papers that we have read for selection of this book chapter. The majority of papers (66) were excluded as they were not relevant and 16 papers were found relevant to answer our research review question. Eleven papers were from the studies that conducted and published in data the selected data bases. Five papers were selected from grey literature, such as reports from Non-governmental organisation, newspapers, reports from districts and radio interviews, to extract stories from community members who experienced constraints to maintaining hygienic conditions during Covid-19. Thematic analysis was used to analyse the results for this book chapter.

3. Results and discussion

The findings that emanated from the literature reviewed regarding the constraints that affected community members' compliance to Covid-19 preventive measures were grouped into two themes. The first theme was insufficient infrastructure, and the sub-themes were overcrowding in informal settlements, lack of running water and poor sanitation. The second theme was poverty as a barrier to hand hygiene during Covid-19 and the sub-themes were affordability of purchasing hand sanitisers and risk factors to illness due to the use of home-made and fake hand sanitisers.

3.1 Overcrowding

Proper housing has always been a challenge in South Africa. This has culminated in the proliferation of informal settlements which are mostly seen in urban areas of South Africa. Those living in inhospitable housing conditions like shacks, were reported to have found the Covid-19 lockdown regulations unbearable. The regulation of social distancing was difficult and impossible to adhere to as those living in crowded households (six people and more), were reported not to have been able to self-isolate where necessary, as they could not keep the necessary distance from one another. The possibility of contracting the Covid-19 infection in such conditions was high.

"As you can see, we live in a dense community and there is little we can do. Many of us live in small shacks in families of 10 to 15, so there is no way we can adhere to the social distance that the government speaks of" [10].

This assertion of poor housing and poverty in general, are considered to have exposed the vulnerable to the worst effects of the Covid-19 pandemic, compared to those who are relatively well-off [11]. Ironically, the inability of the shack-dwellers to comply with the health and safety guidelines or the Covid-19 lockdown restrictions were regarded by many as an unwillingness to conform [11]. Furthermore, the literature review indicated that most shacks in South Africa are built of boards and corrugated iron sheets, less than one meter apart and poorly ventilated due to small windows [12]. Therefore, people living in shacks often do not have a room to relax in but only one room to sleep, which aggravates the spread of infectious diseases.

3.2 Lack of running water

Lack of running water was reported as one of the constraints that contributed to the failure of community members of informal settlements to comply to hand hygiene as a preventive measure to Covid-19. This was supported by the Asivikelane community group in South Africa who reported that in February 2021 "water supply in informal settlements have deteriorated all over the country" [13]. There was a contract for filling water tanks to enable people living in informal settlements to have water. Lack of an adequate water supply to the informal settlements in South Africa, forced people to wake up early to stand in long queues waiting for the delivery of water by tankers. Similarly, De Groot and Lemanski reported that people from informal settlements were saying that.

"Every morning you've got to stand up early so that you could fill up your water bottles/buckets because you only get a certain amount of water per day" [14].

In those circumstances, issues of prioritising hand hygiene were compromised. In those queues, the issue of social distancing was not possible. Socio-Economic Rights Institute of South Africa (SERI) reported that access to water in informal settlements is generally limited to communal water sources [15]. A lack of adequate water supply has been a problem even before Covid-19. This was reported in 2011 when it was shown that about 12% of the 1,068,572 households in the City of Cape Town relied on a communal stand for access to tap water [15]. The number provided of standpipes were fewer than people's need for water. For example, in the Marikana informal settlement, the City of Cape Town has provided 50 communal standpipes to provide water to at least 60,000 residents [15]. Some of the informal settlements used bath water that remained after bathing to wash their hands. In those situations, touching surfaces in their dwellings without washing their hands and further touching their eyes and mouth often resulted in the transmission of infection. Although they wanted to comply circumstances beyond their control became a challenge which was reported as follows:

"How can they tell us to was our hands when we do not have the facilities or the resources to do so? Some informal settlements do not have access to water. And too many are struggling with slow water pressure and not enough working pipes" [16].

Homeless people were also affected by the lack of adhering to hand hygiene and maintaining aseptic techniques despite being moved to tents for shelter during the era of Covid-19. According to Hara, Ncube and Sibanda, a homeless community that was moved to a temporary tented shelter in Cape Town, South Africa, expressed the lack of water as the major challenge [17]. One resident explained that while they were grateful for the tents, they still did not have access to water for hygienic purposes. In those communities, health care workers who were allocated to work with communities who were homeless and those living in informal settlements, were also affected as they could not practice hand hygiene and aseptic techniques because of lack of water. This is illustrated by the following quotations:

> *"The message from our government has been clear: 'Wash your hands!' But those of us living in informal settlements ask ourselves: 'With what?" [16].*

3.3 Poor sanitation

Poor sanitation also came up as one of the constraints due to unavailability of proper toilet facilities and to poor disposal of wastes. Many families in informal settlements are allocated to use one toilet which may not be suitable for the number of people utilising such toilet. In such cases, it sometimes becomes difficult to wait in a queue. People resort to using other methods such as buckets, plastic bags and porta-potties. These practices further exacerbated the poor waste disposal practices and the inability to wash hands after relieving themselves as water is often not available thus exposing them to the spread of the Covid-19 infection.

"we have a challenge – scarcity of water, and that makes it difficult for us to fight the disease. Many in informal settlements have to share a single communal tap" [10].

Furthermore, the use of open fields in which to relieve themselves was found to be causing pollution of the environment. Muanda, Goldin and Haldenwang revealed that informal settlement dwellers use these practices due to poor sanitation that exist in their surroundings, making if difficult for them to wash hands as required, because of lack of water availability [18]. The residents in Khayelitsha protested to the government saying that they cannot practice handwashing because of inadequate water supply as evidenced by the following statement: "'Wash your hands!' But those of us living in informal settlements ask ourselves: 'With what?'" [16].

"Our areas are not regularly cleaned. Even our communal toilets have not been cleaned in over three months, and that could also lead to health issues" [16].

4. Poverty as barrier to hand hygiene during Covid-19

The second theme of this book chapter is poverty as a barrier to hand hygiene during Covid-19 and the sub-themes are affordability of hand sanitisers and the risk factors to illness due to home-made and fake sanitisers.

4.1 Affordability of hand sanitisers

Poverty was found to be a far more important barrier to lockdown regulations and compliance to Covid-19 preventive measures as many people living in informal settlements or shacks were not formally employed [12]. According to Nyashanu,

Simbanegavi and Gibson, people living in shacks or informal settlements depend on the informal sector to support their families [19]. Those people who were selling on the streets could not continue selling their vegetables, fruits, fat cakes and braiding hair to generate an income. In addition, people were expected to buy hand sanitisers as another method to maintain hand hygiene as part of Covid-19 preventative measures.

Supply issues and the high cost of commercially produced sanitisers severely limit the use of Alcohol Based Hand Rubs (ABHRs) in developing countries [20, 21]. This was also the case in South Africa because most people residing in informal settlements could not afford to buy hand sanitisers. The government had to step in and support people living in informal settlements by giving them the hand sanitisers. The KwaZuluNatal (KZN) Provincial Executive Council directed the Human Settlements Department to launch an intensive sanitisation programme in informal settlements to assist them with hand sanitizers [10]. The sanitisation programme was implemented in all 729 informal settlements in the province's 10 district municipalities and eThekwini Metro in April 2020 where bars of soap and hand sanitisers were distributed to households [10].

However, people living in informal settlements in Cape Town felt that the South African Government did not pay much attention to their needs when it comes to maintaining hand hygiene practices during Covid-19. In support of this, more than 80% of residents in Cape Town's informal settlements said they had not received soap or hand sanitiser from the government [22]. One of the residents in informal settlements in South Africa said:

> *"Where are we supposed to get money for sanitisers when we don't work?" [16].*
>
> *"That is for rich people who can afford to buy soap all the time. Hand sanitiser is but a pipe dream. With little to no funds to secure basic necessities, hand sanitiser and extra soap are luxuries" [10].*

"How are we supposed to get money for sanitiser when we don't work?" We need money to buy bread for the children who are now staying at home for longer periods [23]."

Most of the residents in informal settlements rely on social grants. One of the residents in informal settlements raised this issue in a form of question and said:

"They barely meet our daily needs; why can't the government go around to communities like ours and at the very least provide us with gloves, masks, and sanitisers during this period? [23]."

As much as the government tried to provide for sanitisers to reach everyone in need, the issue of inequality played a big role as the municipalities did not have enough money and equal resources for distribution.

4.2 Risk factors to illness due to the use of home-made and fake hand sanitisers

South Africans were not exempt from the use of fake hand sanitisers. The demand for hand sanitisers was high during the Covid-19 era, therefore some companies ended up making fake sanitisers [24]. The use of substandard and fake hand sanitisers was found to be dangerous to uninformed consumers because they cause skin irritant health related problems [24]. Also, Perera reported that knowledge on the use the use of fake hand sanitisers could pose a greater risk among residents in informal settlements in South Africa. There is a need for creating health awareness regarding the use of fake hand sanitisers for people in informal settlement [25].

Some of the measures that were used by people were home-made hand sanitisers. For example, In South Africa, people would say:

> *"We combine household disinfectant cleaning solutions such as Jik, Sunlight dishwashing solution, and/or Domestos to use as hand sanitisers and disinfectant for the prevention of Covid-19."*

In support of this, people in developed countries were also using home-made disinfectant for prevention of Covid-19 [26]. However, it has been reported that the 'misuse' of home-based hand sanitisers resulted in poisoning which was typically centred on chemicals used for cleaning at home in the era of Covid-19 [27].

5. Conclusion

The living conditions of people in informal settlements made it difficult for them to adhere to Covid-19 regulations in South Africa. Overcrowding was one of the challenges that was experienced by people living in informal settlements because as there was no enough space to maintain social distancing, self-isolation and quarantine when the need arose. This was exacerbated by the lack of access to running water for people to practice hand hygiene, as required. Lack of running water resulted in poor sanitation as people could not flush their toilets and wash to maintain hand hygiene. The majority of people in informal settlements were working in firms that closed and some of them had informal businesses which could not run as usual due to lockdown regulations. Some people decided to make their own home-based sanitizers, while on the other hand companies produced fake hand sanitisers which had a negative impact on their integumentary system resulting to skin rashes and cracks and predisposing them to poisoning. WASH is an important strategy to promote hygiene and to prevent the spread of infectious disease. The communities must be taught about hand washing as a basic course that is taught from the schools in order to attain goal 3 and 6. The South African government must made efforts to provide housing, better access to water and improve sanitation.

Author details

Fhumulani M. Mulaudzi, Nombulelo V. Sepeng*, Ndivhaleni R. Lavhelani and Tintswalo V. Nesengani
Faculty of Health Sciences, Department of Nursing Sciences, University of Pretoria, Tshwane, South Africa

*Address all correspondence to: nombulelo.sepeng@up.ac.za

References

[1] Adhikari SP, Meng S, Wu YJ, Mao YP, Ye RX, Wang QZ, et al. Epidemiology, causes, clinical manifestation and diagnosis, prevention and control of coronavirus disease (COVID-19) during the early outbreak period: A scoping review. Infectious Diseases of Poverty. 2020;**9**(1):1-2

[2] Rundle CW, Presley CL, Militello M, Barber C, Powell DL, Jacob SE, et al. Hand hygiene during COVID-19: Recommendations from the American contact dermatitis society. Journal of the American Academy of Dermatology. 2020;**83**(6):1730-1737

[3] World Health Organization. Hygiene: UN-Water GLAAS Findings on National Policies, Plans, Targets and Finance. Geneva: World Health Organization; 2020 Licence: CC BY-NC-SA 3.0 IGO

[4] UNICEF. State of the World's Sanitation: An Urgent Call to Transform Sanitation for Better Health, Environments, Economies and Societies. New York: United Nations Children's Fund (UNICEF) and the World Health Organization; 2020

[5] Chetty S, Bangalee V. Lessons from COVID-19 in South Africa: Keeping our environment clean should be the first law of health. South African Family Practice. 2021;**63**(1):1-3

[6] United Nations. Transforming our world: The 2030 agenda for sustainable development. Available from: https://sustainabledevelopment.un.org/content/documents/21252030%20agenda%20for%20sustainable%20development%20web.pdf. [Accessed: August 19, 2022)

[7] Strategic plan for the fiscal years. 2020. 2021 to 2024, 25, Department of Water and Sanitation. Available from: https://www.dws.gov.za/documents/Other/Strategic%20Plan/2021/Strategic%20Plan%202020-21%20to%202024-25_23Mar2020.pdf. [Accessed: July 10, 2022]

[8] Haddout S, Priya KL, Hoguane AM, Ljubenkov I. Water scarcity: A big challenge to slums in Africa to fight against COVID-19. Science & Technology Libraries. 2020;**39**(3):281-288

[9] Anim DO, Ofori-Asenso R. Water scarcity and COVID-19 in sub-Saharan Africa. Journal of Infection. 2020;**81**(2):e108-e109

[10] Sokanyile. Hand sanitiser and social distancing not priorities in communities battling poverty. 2022. Available from: https://www.iol.co.za/news/south-africa/western-cape/hand-sanitiser-and-social-distancing-not-priorities-in-communities-battling-poverty-45322784. [Accessed: August 18, 2022]

[11] Nwosu CO, Oyenubi A. Income-related health inequalities associated with the coronavirus pandemic in South Africa: A decomposition analysis. International Journal for Equity in Health. 2021;**20**(1):1-2

[12] Jansen J, Madhi SA. How to do social distancing in a shack: COVID-19 in the south African context. South African Journal of Science. 2022;**118**(5-6):1-3

[13] Asivikelane (let's protect one another): voices of informal settlement residents during the Covid-19 crisis. Available from: http://www.asivikelane.org.za/. [Accessed: August 22, 2022]

[14] De Groot J, Lemanski C. COVID-19 responses: Infrastructure inequality and

privileged capacity to transform everyday life in South Africa. Environment and Urbanization. 2021;**33**(1):255-272

[15] Socio-Economic Rights Institute of South Africa (SERI). Informal Settlements and Human Rights in South Africa. Available from: https://www.ohchr.org/sites/default/files/Documents/Issues/Housing/InformalSettlements/SERI.pdf. [Accessed: August 22, 2022]

[16] Nombembe P. 'Wash your hands - with what?' – Cape Town shack dwellers protest over water a day before lockdown. TimesLive; Available from: https://www.timeslive.co.za/news/south-africa/2020-03-25-wash-your-hands-with-what-cape-town-shack-dwellers-protest-over-water-a-day-before-lockdown/. [Accessed: August 22, 2022]

[17] Hara M, Ncube B, Sibanda D. Water and Sanitation in the Face of Covid-19 in Cape Town's Townships and Informal Settlements. Cape Town, South Africa: Institute for Poverty, Land and Agrarian Studies (PLAAS), University of the Western Cape (UWC); 2020. p. 5

[18] Muanda C, Goldin J, Haldenwang R. Factors and impacts of informal settlements residents' sanitation practices on access and sustainability of sanitation services in the policy context of free basic sanitation. Journal of Water, Sanitation and Hygiene for Development. 2020;**10**(2):238-248

[19] Nyashanu M, Simbanegavi P, Gibson L. Exploring the impact of COVID-19 pandemic lockdown on informal settlements in Tshwane Gauteng Province, South Africa. Global Public Health. 2020;**15**(10):1443-1453

[20] Allegranzi B, Pittet D. Healthcare-associated infection in developing countries: Simple solutions to meet complex challenges. Infection Control & Hospital Epidemiology. 2007;**28**(12):1323-1327

[21] Pittet D, Allegranzi B, Storr J, Nejad SB, Dziekan G, Leotsakos A, et al. Infection control as a major World Health Organization priority for developing countries. Journal of hospital infection. 2008;**68**(4):285-292

[22] Brief 2. Asivikelane Let's Protect One Another: Voices Of Informal Settlement Residents During The Covid-19 Crisis. 2020. Available from: https://asivikelane.org/wp-content/uploads/2020/12/brief-2-access-to-basic-sanitation-during-covid-19-in-the-coct.pdf. [Accessed August 18, 2022]

[23] South African Government. Let's grow South Africa Together: KwaZulu-Natal launches Coronavirus COVID 19 informal settlements sanitisation programme. Available from: https://www.gov.za/speeches/kwazulu-natal-launches-coronavirus-covid-19-informal-settlements-sanitisation-programme-21. [Accessed: August 18, 2022]

[24] Govender K, Mdanda S, Baijnath S, Kruger HG, Govender T, Naicker T. The analysis of alcohol content in hand sanitisers (in the Durban region) using gas chromatography-mass spectrometry during the COVID-19 pandemic. South African Journal of Chemistry. 2022;**76**:20-24

[25] Perera M. Is there any commonality between transmition of antimicrobial resistant genes and alcohol tolerant genes from one bacterium to another?. Academia Letters. 2021:2

[26] Moskowitz R. How to make disinfectant wipes at home. 2020. Available from: reviewed.com

[27] Cook MA, Brooke N. Event-based surveillance of poisonings and potentially hazardous exposures over 12 months of the COVID-19 pandemic. International journal of environmental research and public health. 2021;**18**(21):11133

Chapter 5

Air Pollution Monitoring and Its Health Impact in Belarus

Nadzeya Dziarzhynskaya, Larisa Hindziuk and Andrey Hindziuk

Abstract

The chapter contains information on the state of air pollution in the Republic of Belarus and Minsk, including emissions and concentrations of pollutants. Organization of air quality monitoring system overviews monitoring network and monitoring posts, list of controlled substances, frequency, and organization of sampling. The chapter contains applied methods for evaluating the results of laboratory monitoring of atmospheric air pollution, and complex indicators are used to assess the degree of atmospheric pollution. The main results of studies of the impact of atmospheric air pollution in the Republic of Belarus on the state of public health conducted during the last 20 years will be discussed.

Keywords: atmospheric air, pollution, monitoring system, public health

1. Introduction

Atmospheric air is a significant component of the human environment and has a multi-vector impact on human health, which can be realized both directly by inhaling atmospheric air and due to the migration of harmful substances from the atmosphere into soil, water, and accumulation in food. At the individual level, the time a person spends outdoors largely determines the degree of influence of atmospheric air on health. However, at the population level, despite the professional and age affiliation, the state of the atmospheric air is in second place after socioeconomic factors in the structure of economic losses in the gross domestic product of developed countries from mortality and morbidity of the population associated with the negative impact of environmental factors [1].

According to the World Health Organization, air pollution is the most important environmental risk factor for public health in the European Region [2]. An increase in the degree of atmospheric air pollution (ceteris paribus) is manifested by an increase in the incidence of acute respiratory infections in the population by 6–7% due to nonspecific influence [3].

At the same time, large contingents of the population of cities are exposed to atmospheric pollution, where the degree of atmospheric air pollution is characterized by a multicomponent and dynamic composition. The amount of chemicals in the atmospheric air of populated areas reaches several tens, sometimes hundreds [3–6].

Assessment of atmospheric air quality in settlements and its impact on the health of the population are widely used to make urban planning decisions with the active growth of settlements, the construction and reconstruction of industrial enterprises, and the expansion of residential development through the use of the territory adjacent to enterprises and other facilities.

2. Methods

2.1 Analytical laboratory control

Methods of analytical laboratory control are used in the study of the degree of air pollution in the Republic of Belarus on the basis of data obtained from the following sources:

- stationary observation posts of the Republican Center for Radiation Control and Environmental Monitoring of the Ministry of Natural Resources and Environmental Protection of the Republic of Belarus,
- route posts of institutions of the Ministry of Health of the Republic of Belarus, carrying out state sanitary supervision, and
- mobile (under-torch) posts (industrial control).

2.1.1 Stationary posts

Stationary posts are observation points of the National Environmental Monitoring System of the Republic of Belarus, included in the State Register of observation points of the Republic of Belarus. The Ministry of Natural Resources and Environmental Protection of the Republic of Belarus coordinates the work in the field of atmospheric air monitoring. At present, monitoring of the state of atmospheric air is carried out in 19 industrial cities of the republic, including regional centers—**Figure 1**.

There are 67 stationary posts installed in the cities [7]. In Minsk—12 stations, in Mahilyow, Homiel, and Vitsebsk—5 each, in Brest and Hrodna—4 each; in other

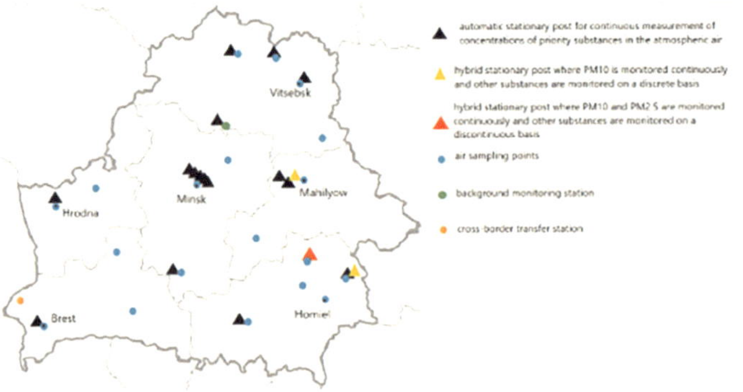

Figure 1.
Location of stationary observation posts of the Republican Center for Radiation Control and Environmental Monitoring.

industrial centers—1–3 stations. Regular observations cover the territories where almost 87% of the population of large- and medium-sized cities of the republic lives. In all cities, the concentrations of the main pollutants are determined:

- particulate matter (undifferentiated dust/aerosol),
- sulfur dioxide,
- carbon monoxide, and
- nitrogen dioxide.

Concentrations of priority-specific pollutants are also measured:

- formaldehyde,
- ammonia,
- phenol,
- hydrogen sulfide, and
- carbon disulfide.

When choosing a priority list of specific substances, emissions of each substance (data from the National Statistical Committee of the Republic of Belarus), the size of the city, maximum allowable concentrations, and dispersion coefficients are taken into account. In all controlled cities, the content of lead and cadmium in the air is determined, in 16 cities—benz/a/pyrene, in 9 cities—hydrocarbons. Automatic stations measure concentrations of PM_{10} and ground-level ozone. Measurements of the concentrations of $PM_{2.5}$ microns in size are carried out in Minsk (the area of Geroev 120 Divizii St.) and Zhlobin (the area of Prigorodnaya St.) [7].

Stationary posts are designed to obtain information on maximum and average daily concentrations. Observations of the state of atmospheric air in a discrete mode are carried out daily on working days, at 1, 7, 13, and 19 hours (air samples are taken by a technician into absorption devices or aerosol filters for 20 minutes and delivered to the laboratory, where the subsequent chemical analysis is carried out). At automatic stationary posts, measurements are carried out by continuous sampling, during all day and night. Air quality is determined by several thousand measurements per year.

2.1.2 Route posts

Route posts carry out air quality control as part of the state sanitary supervision of institutions of the Ministry of Health of the Republic of Belarus. Route post is designed for regular air sampling when it is not possible (not feasible) to establish a stationary post or it is necessary to study the state of air pollution in certain areas, for example, in new residential areas. Observations at route posts are carried out using a mobile laboratory, which is equipped with the necessary instruments. One car attends around 4–5 points per working day. The order in which the vehicle goes around the selected waypoints should be the same in order to ensure that the concentrations of impurities are determined at the same time. Route posts are located in places selected on the basis of a mandatory preliminary study of urban air pollution by industrial emissions, vehicle emissions, and other sources and the study of meteorological conditions for the dispersion of impurities through episodic observations. Posts must be installed first of all in those residential areas where the highest average levels of pollution are possible, then in the administrative center of the settlement and in residential areas with various types of buildings, as well as in parks and recreation areas. The most polluted areas include zones of the highest maximum one-time and average daily concentrations created by emissions from industrial enterprises, as well as motor transport routes. At the route posts, the content of specific impurities of the priority list, characteristic of nearby emission sources, is monitored. For example, in Minsk list of chemicals includes the following:

- acrolein,
- benzene,
- 1,3—butadiene,
- particulate matter (undifferentiated dust/aerosol),
- sulfur dioxide,
- nitrogen dioxide,
- carbon monoxide,
- phenol,
- xylene, and
- formaldehyde.

Considering the variety of substances present in the air of the city, this list allows us to focus on the most dangerous pollutants for health, which are subject to control in the first place.

The duration of air sampling at route posts for determining maximum concentrations of impurities is 20–30 minutes, and sampling is made few times per month. Further, air samples are delivered to the laboratory, where a chemical study of air samples is carried out, then the data are sent for further analysis.

2.1.3 Mobile (under-torch) posts

Mobile (under-torch) posts carry out industrial control of air pollution. A mobile (under-torch) post is designed for sampling under a smoke (gas) torch in order to identify the zone of influence of a source of industrial emissions. Observations under the torch of the enterprise are also carried out with the help of an equipped car. During a work shift (8 hours), one machine can carry out observations at 8–10 points. Mobile posts are points located at fixed distances from the source. They move in accordance with the direction of the torch of the surveyed emission source (according to wind direction).

To determine the maximum concentrations of pollutants that are created by emissions from enterprises to a particular area of the city, as well as the size of the zone of impurity distribution from a given enterprise, under-torch observations are organized, that is, measurements of impurity concentrations under the axis of the plume of emissions from pipes of industrial enterprises. The location of the points where air samples are taken to determine the concentrations of harmful substances varies depending on the direction of the torch. Torch observations are carried out in the area of a separate emission source or a group of sources both within the city and outside it.

Sampling during under-torch observations is carried out at distances of 0.5, 1, 2, 3, 4, 6, 8, 10, 15, and 30 km from the source of pollution on the leeward side of it. More often, observations should be made at distances of 10–40 average pipe heights from the source, where the probability of the appearance of a maximum concentration is especially high. Observations are carried out for specific substances characteristic of a given enterprise. Air sampling under the torch is carried out at a height of 1.5–3.5 m from the ground in accordance with the methodology used for observations at a stationary post. Under-torch observations should be carried out at the time of measurements at stationary and route posts and additionally at other times in order to study the distribution of maximum concentrations at different hours of the day.

2.2 Evaluation of the results of laboratory measurements

After determining the concentrations of polluting chemicals in the atmospheric air, the obtained values are evaluated in accordance with the current hygienic standards [8]. When comparing the obtained concentrations with their hygienic standards, it is necessary to comply with the averaging periods—the maximum acute concentrations are compared with the values of the maximum standards, the average daily—with the average daily, etc. In Republic of Belarus, there are three types of standards maximum acute, average daily, and average annual.

Assessment taking into account the effect of the summation of the harmful effects of pollutants is also made. After assessing the content of individual pollutants in the atmospheric air, it is necessary to check whether they have a summation effect in accordance with **Table 3** of the Hygiene Standard [8]. With the simultaneous content in the atmospheric air of several pollutants with the effect of summation, the sum of the ratios of the actual concentrations of each of them in the air to their standards should not exceed one (Eq. (1)):

$$\frac{C}{Stndr} + \frac{C_1}{Stndr_1} + \dots + \frac{C_n}{Stndr_n} \le 1 \quad (1)$$

where.

$C, C_1 \dots C_n$ are concentrations of pollutants with the summation effect, μg/m^3.

$Stndr, Stndr_1 \dots Stndr_n$ are the values of hygienic standards for pollutants with the summation effect, μg/m^3.

The assessment of the joint content of polluting chemicals in the atmospheric air, taking into account the effects of summation, is carried out only if the pollution contains all the substances included in the summation group. If at least one substance is missing, then it is considered that the summation group has not formed, and the assessment is not carried out.

The above hygiene standards (both for individual substances and for summation groups) are legally valid—if they are exceeded, measures must be taken to reduce the content of pollutants.

2.3 Complex indicators of atmospheric pollution

2.3.1 Complex indicator P

Hygienic assessment of the degree of atmospheric air pollution with the simultaneous presence of several pollutants in Belarus is carried out according to the value of the "P" indicator, which takes into account the multiplicity of exceeding the hygiene standard, the hazard class of the substance, and the amount of chemical substances present in the atmospheric air together.

Complex indicator "P" represents atmospheric air as a dynamic environment with a certain general level of pollution that has a diverse impact on the health of the population, which makes it possible not to study separately the processes of exposure to each of the pollutants. This method takes into account the combined action of pollutants according to the type of incomplete summation.

Calculation of the complex indicator "P" is carried out according to the following formula Eq. (2):

$$\mathbf{P_i = \sum_{i=1}^{n} K_i^2} \tag{2}$$

where

K_i is isoefficiency concentrations of pollutants, which are calculated according to the following Eq. (3):

$$\mathbf{K_i = \left(\frac{C}{Stndr}\right) * i} \tag{3}$$

where.

C is concentration of pollutant, μg/m^3,

Stndr is value of hygienic standard for pollutant, μg/m^3, and

i is isoefficiency coefficient that depends on substance hazard class:

- 1st class—2;
- 2nd class—1.5;
- 3rd class—1; and
- 4th class—0.8.

Hygienic assessment of the degree of atmospheric air pollution by a complex of pollutants is carried out in accordance with **Table 1**.

The first degree is safe for the health of the population, with pollution of the II–V degree, and the frequency of adverse effects increases with an increase in the degree of atmospheric pollution—**Table 2**.

It should be noted that the complex indicator P has no legal force (the measures indicated in the tables are advisory in nature) and is more often used in scientific research or when comparing territories with a heterogeneous composition of atmospheric air pollution.

Degree of atmospheric air pollution	Value of complex indicator "P" with the number atmospheric pollutants			
	2–3 pollutants	4–9 pollutants	10–20 pollutants	21 and more pollutants
I—admissible	Up to 1.6	Up to 3	Up to 5	Up to 7.1
II—weak	1.7–3.2	3.1–4.8	5.1–6.4	7.2–8
III—moderate	3.3–6.4	4.9–9.6	6.5–12.8	8.1–16
IV—strong	6.5–12.8	9.7–19.2	12.9–25.6	16.1–32
V—dangerous	12.9 and more	19.3 and more	25.7 and more	32.1 and more

Table 1.
Hygienic assessment of the degree of atmospheric air pollution by the complex of pollutants.

Degree of atmospheric air pollution	Prognosed risk level	Prognosed gradations of population health	Measures to be taken
I—admissible	1: 10000000 (10^{-7}; E-07), acceptable risk level	Adaptation (baseline incidence)	Low priority. The current risk management system is sufficient. No additional measures required
II—weak	1: 1000000 (10^{-6}; E-06), acceptable risk level	Compensation/resistance (baseline incidence)	Low priority. The current risk management system is sufficient. No additional measures required
III—moderate	1: 100000 (10^{-5}; E-05), risk is considered high enough	Adaptation stress (significant excess of baseline incidence)	Medium priority. Hazard identification and risk mitigation decisions
IV—strong	1: 10000 (10^{-4}; E-04), risk is assessed as unacceptable	Overstrain of adaptation (significant excess of the highest limit of the baseline incidence)	High priority. Hazard identification, health risk assessment studies and simultaneous implementation of emergency risk reduction measures
V—dangerous	1: 1000 (10^{-3}; E-03), risk is assessed as unallowable	Disruption of adaptation (exceeding baseline incidence by several times)	High priority. Urgent adoption of a set of emergency measures to reduce the risk

Table 2.
Prognosed gradations of population health and risk levels depending on the degree of atmospheric air pollution.

2.3.2 Complex air pollution index

Complex air pollution index (CAPI) is a quantitative measure of the level of air pollution created by several chemicals present in the atmosphere of a city. The index allows us to present an integral level of air pollution in the city with one number. When calculating complex air pollution index, as a rule, data on the main five substances are used, which make the maximum contribution to the level of atmospheric air pollution in the territory under consideration.

$CAPI_5$	Level of atmospheric pollution
≤ 5	Low
6 < CAPI ≤8	Average
9 ≤ CAPI <15	Above average
CAPI >15	Well above average

Table 3.
Level of atmospheric pollution by the value of $CAPI_5$.

Calculation of complex air pollution index is carried out according to the following formula (Eq. (4)):

$$CAPI = \sum_{k=5}^{n} \left(\frac{C}{Stndr} \right)^{i} \tag{4}$$

where C is concentration of pollutant, μg/m^3,
Stndr is value of hygienic standard for pollutant, μg/m^3, and
i is isoefficiency coefficient that depends on substance hazard class:

- 1st class—1.7;
- 2nd class—1.3;
- 3rd class—1; and
- 4th class—0.9.

Usually, complex air pollution index is calculated for all pollutants, and then, it is necessary to determine five main ones that make the maximum contribution to the value of complex air pollution index. The resulting value is denoted by index 5 ($CAPI_5$) and can be used to compare the level of air pollution in different areas, regardless of which five substances are included in this indicator. Assessment of the level of atmospheric pollution by the value of $CAPI_5$ is carried out in accordance with **Table 3**.

Complex air pollution index also has no legal force; in case of obtaining high values, preventive measures to reduce the concentrations of pollutants can only be advisory in nature. In addition, in contrast to the complex indicator P, there is no scale for CAPI that allows us to predict possible effects on population health. This indicator is more often accepted in the ecological field and also allows us to compare areas with different compositions of atmospheric pollution.

3. Results

3.1 Air pollution sources in Belarus

The entry of pollutants into the atmospheric air occurs as a result of the activity of natural and anthropogenic sources, as well as a result of the regional and transboundary transfer. Of the greatest interest among these sources are anthropogenic, as they make a significant contribution to the formation of atmospheric air pollution and are also the most accessible for correction and development of preventive measures.

According to the Ministry of Natural Resources and Environmental Protection [5], the National Statistical Committee [6], the share of emissions from stationary sources is about 38.5% of total emissions from all sources in the territory of the Republic of Belarus—**Figure 2**.

In addition, there is a tendency to reduce both the total amount of emissions into the atmospheric air from stationary and mobile sources. Geographically, the largest share of emissions was registered in Minsk region, Brest region, and Vitsebsk region—**Figure 3**.

The composition of emissions from pollution sources by substances as of 2020 was presented by carbon monoxide (46.98% of emissions), hydrocarbons (30.23%),

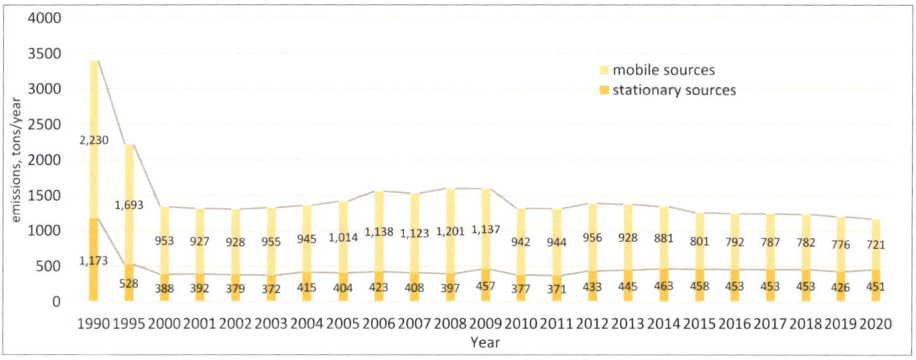

Figure 2.
Dynamics of emissions into the atmospheric air of the Republic of Belarus from stationary and mobile sources in 1990–2020.

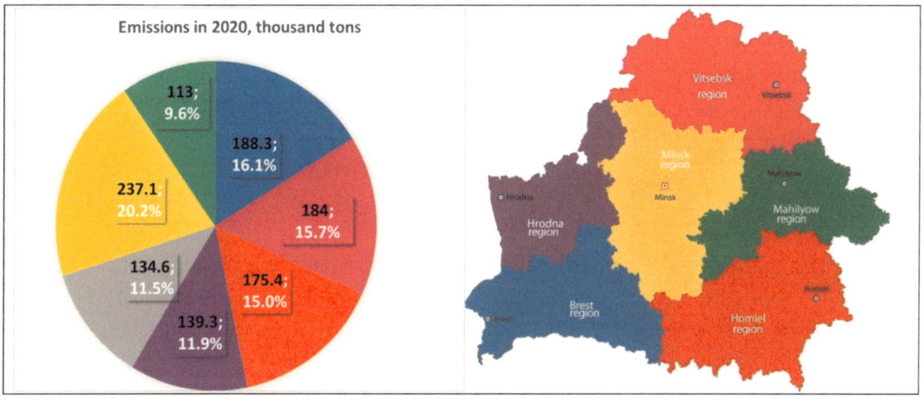

Figure 3.
Emissions of harmful substances into the atmospheric air in regions of the Republic of Belarus from stationary and mobile sources in 2020.

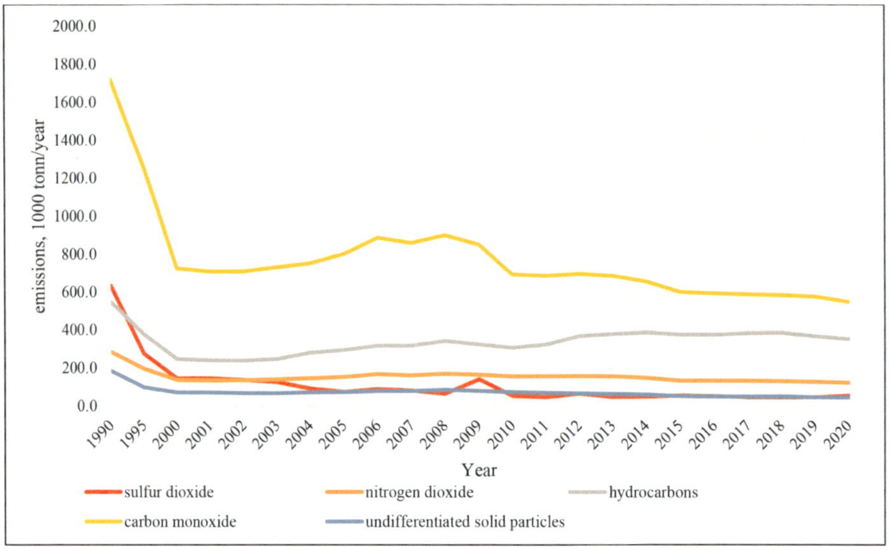

Figure 4.
Dynamics of emissions of harmful substances into the atmospheric air of the Republic of Belarus from stationary and mobile sources in 1990–2020.

nitrogen dioxide (10.65%), sulfur dioxide (4.81%), and particulate matter (undifferentiated dust/aerosol) (3.96%)—**Figure 4**.

At the same time, 99.82% of emissions of sulfur dioxide and 84.85% of carbon monoxide were formed due to stationary sources, and 64.02% of emissions of nitrogen dioxide, 57.17% of hydrocarbons, and 52.16% of undifferentiated solid particles were formed due to stationary sources.

Data on the quantitative and qualitative composition of emissions from stationary sources are formed on the basis of information provided by enterprises in the form of statistical reporting. By 2020, the main share of emissions was accounted for agriculture, forestry and fisheries (34.2%), manufacturing industry (33.8%), and electricity generation (21.4%). The largest contribution in the manufacturing industry was made by oil refining (43.1%). The qualitative composition of emissions from stationary sources is diverse and varies significantly depending on the characteristics of the technological process of the facility. Despite the fact that the contribution of emissions from stationary sources to emissions from all sources is about a third, the adverse effects associated with the operation of these sources are of great importance due to the possibility of releasing hazardous compounds, as well as compounds with long-term effects (carcinogenesis, teratogenicity, embryotoxicity, etc.). The distribution and dispersion of emissions from stationary sources depend on many conditions: the temperature of the ejected air jet, the height of the source of emission, the climatic and meteorological characteristics of the area. These indicators are constant for each stationary source of emissions, which makes it easier to predict the spread of pollutants and allows to develop effective measures to reduce the adverse impact of released chemicals on public health.

The share of emissions from mobile sources in 2020 was 61.5% in the composition of gross emissions from all sources on the territory of the Republic of Belarus [6]. The value of gross emissions from mobile sources is determined by the calculation method based on specific emission indicators per unit of fuel used for generalized groups of vehicles and environmental classes, as well as data on the volume of fuel consumed for transport operations [6]. The largest number of emissions from mobile sources falls on the city of Minsk and the Minsk region, and Grodno regions [5]. The qualitative composition of emissions from mobile sources is relatively constant and is represented by carbon monoxide, hydrocarbons, nitrogen oxides, particulate matter, and sulfur oxides. The distribution and dispersion of emissions from mobile sources are also related to the natural, climatic, and meteorological characteristics of the area; however, it is more difficult to predict the real impact of emissions from mobile sources on public health due to the variable number of emission sources and the time of their operation.

Thus, the qualitative and quantitative composition of atmospheric air pollution in the Republic of Belarus is due to the anthropogenic effect of stationary and mobile sources of emissions. There is a constant collection and processing of information on the composition and amount of chemicals emitted into the atmospheric air, the

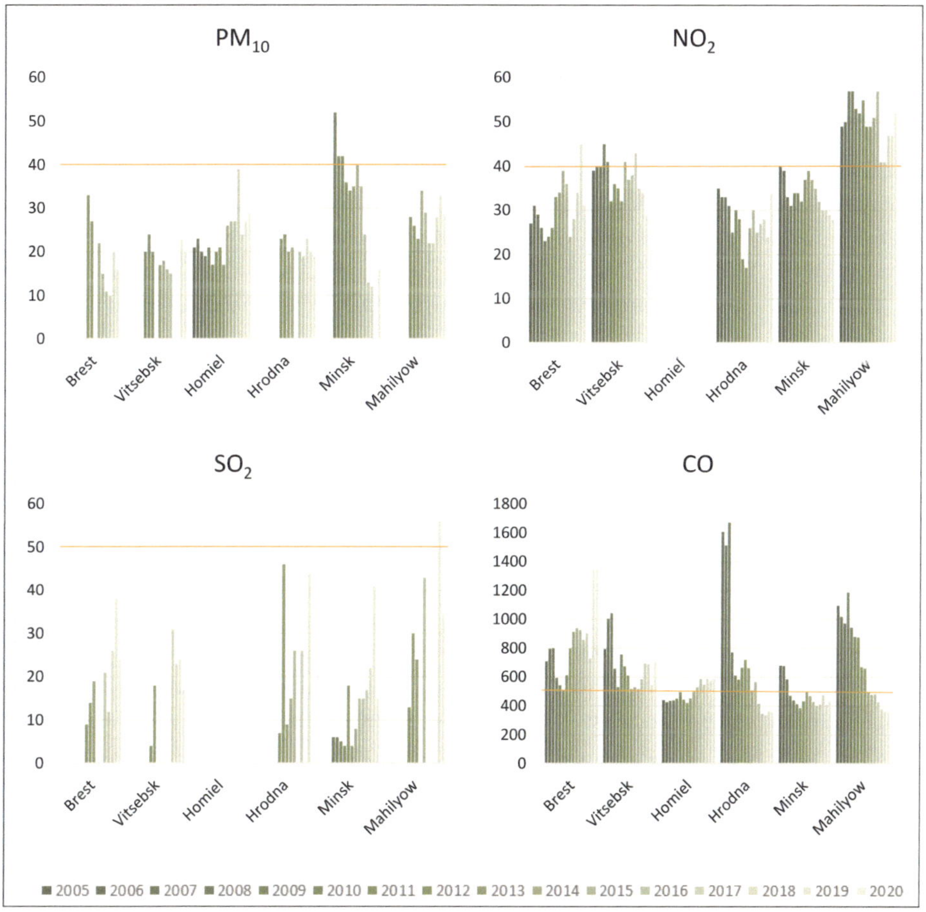

Figure 5.
*Annual concentrations in μg/m³ of PM10, NO2, SO2, CO from stationary observation posts in biggest cities for period 2005–2020.*In some cases, there were no average annual concentration, since measurements were not carried out or there were not enough of them to calculate the average daily concentration.*Red line marks annual level of hygienic standard for pollutant.*

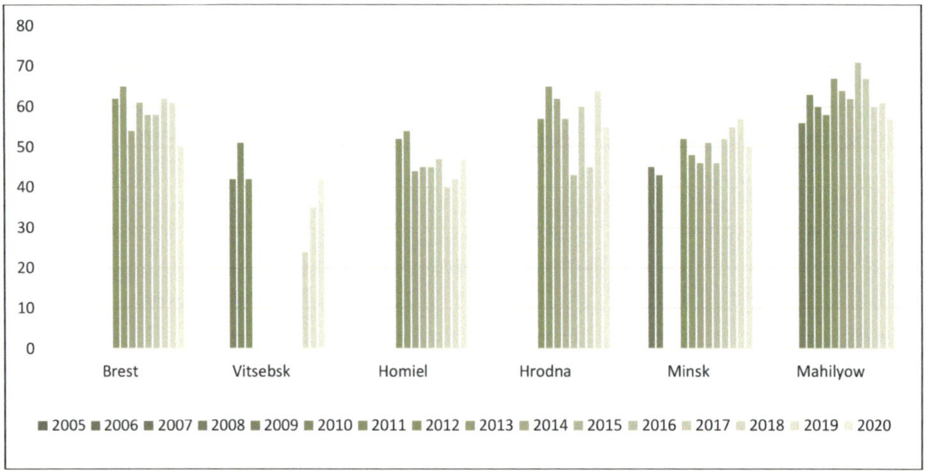

Figure 6.
*Annual concentrations in μg/m³ of tropospheric ozone from stationary observation posts in biggest cities for period 2005–2020.*In some cases, there were no average annual concentration, since measurements were not carried out or there were not enough of them to calculate the average daily concentration.*

territorial distribution of sources, and their contribution to the value of gross emissions from all sources. In most cases, data on the qualitative and quantitative composition of emissions from each source are obtained by calculation.

3.2 Concentrations of pollutants in atmospheric air of Belarus

According to information from stationary observation posts of the Republican Center for Radiation Control and Environmental Monitoring of the Ministry of Natural Resources and Environmental Protection of the Republic of Belarus during period from 2005 to 2020 [5], the following average annual concentrations of the main pollutants in the atmospheric air were recorded in the largest cities of the Republic—**Figure 5**.

As it is seen from **Figure 5**, mostly there was a trend toward a decrease in the content of the main pollutants. Values of the average annual concentrations were obtained by mathematical averaging of the concentrations received from stationary observation posts on a daily basis. Also, daily concentrations of tropospheric ozone were mathematically averaged to the annual concentrations—**Figure 6**.

In all cases, concentrations of tropospheric ozone did not exceed level of hygienic standard. Thus, the level of pollution in large cities of Belarus remains quite intense. However, there has been a downward trend in the concentrations of major pollutants over the past 15 years.

4. Discussion

4.1 Impact of air pollution on health

Impact of air pollution on public health is beyond doubt. An objective quantitative and qualitative assessment of the effects of atmospheric air pollution are difficult due to the heterogeneity and variability of the chemical composition of pollution and physical properties of the environment itself, differences in individual sensitivity of different population groups, the impossibility of excluding the effects of other factors (nutrition, living conditions, professional factors, etc.), and the inability to simulate the impact of the entire air environment in laboratory conditions. In this regard, studies of the effect of polluting chemicals contained in the atmospheric air on the health of the population are represented by a large number of studies of various designs. Among them, the main following results in Belarus can be distinguished:

A group of studies was devoted to studying the effect of hydrocarbons on the state of public health: atmospheric air pollution with hydrocarbons was found to be the cause of a statistically significant increase in incidence rate from 1.5 to 7 times of 19 types of diseases in population: diseases of the upper respiratory tract and respiratory organs, peripheral nervous, cardiovascular system, allergic diseases, and oncological diseases [4].

In Mahilyow, a significant relationship was found between incidence rate of chronic diseases of the tonsils and adenoids, pneumonia, bronchial asthma, and high levels of dust in the atmosphere in the adult population. The same authors studied the content of phenol and formaldehyde in the atmosphere of Homiel and revealed that increased content of pollutants was associated with an increase in the incidence rates of pneumonia in the adult population. Authors also determined the value of complex indicator "P" for some districts of Minsk and established that the actual level of the children incidence rate of bronchial asthma exceeded the calculated indicator based on the regression mathematical model from 0.54 to 2.06 times. A significant relationship was also established between the total air pollution in Minsk and children incidence rates of chronic diseases of the tonsils and adenoids, bronchial asthma, and in Hrodna—chronic pharyngitis [9].

Correlation analysis made by other group of research studies highlighted a positive correlation between asthma incidence rate and concentrations of particulate matter (dust/aerosol undifferentiated in composition), lead, ammonia, and nitrogen dioxide in Minsk [10].

In addition, the issue of the presence and composition of pollen allergens in the atmospheric air of Minsk and the relationship between the content of these allergens and the manifestations of bronchial asthma in children have been studied quite widely and in detail [11].

Dependence of prevalence levels among the population with infections of the upper respiratory tract and value of complex indicator "P" was established, which was described by a linear type equation $y = 218.97 + 12.73x$ ($r = 0.54$, $p = 0.001$). According to the data obtained, an increased value of complex indicator "P" by 1 entails an increase in the prevalence by 12.73 cases per 1000 population. Among studied infections of the upper respiratory environmental conditioning was found for acute nasopharyngitis, pharyngitis, tonsillitis, and bronchitis, as well as for acute respiratory diseases [12].

Using the risk assessment methodology, a group of Belarusian authors calculated health risk levels from air pollution in large cities of Belarus. Performed calculations of the health risk values for the child population showed that high risk of prevalence rates was typical for Vitsebsk and Homiel, an increased one—for Hrodna, Minsk, Mahilyow, and a minimum one for Brest. Among certain diseases, neoplasms, infectious diseases, diseases of the endocrine system, blood and hematopoietic tissues, nervous system, and respiratory organs had a high risk. For adult population, high health risk of incidence rates was recorded for Brest, Vitsebsk, Minsk, and Mahilyow.

It was confirmed that the value of complex indicator "P" is quite consistent with the expected level of health of the population [13].

To date, a sufficiently large amount of data have been accumulated, indicating that air pollution contributes to the formation of the incidence of various diseases all over the world. Thus, the presence of significantly higher incidence rates of myocardial infarction (by 1.43 times) and ischemic cardiomyopathy (by 1.12 times) was found among the population living in the area of major transport routes [14]. An analysis of more than 20 studies of the content of particulate matter of various fractions in the atmospheric air and stroke incidence rates indicates the presence of a statistically significant relationship between these indicators: in the countries of North America and Europe, for every 10 $\mu g/m^3$ increase in the content of particulate matter up to 10 μm, 1.062 times increased risk of stroke [15]. Studies of the degree of air pollution in Ireland showed that the introduction of bans on the burning of coal significantly reduced the incidence of respiratory diseases [16]. Air pollution can lead to an increase in the incidence of noncommunicable diseases among the population, including not only respiratory, but also cardiovascular diseases: hypertension, myocardial infarction, angina pectoris, chronic pharyngitis, chronic bronchitis, and bronchial asthma [17, 18]. At the same time, the incidence rate indicates an already formed reaction in the body to an adverse effect in the form of a disease, which makes it difficult to quickly analyze the level of the adverse effect of the factor and develop effective preventive measures.

The impact of polluted atmospheric air on the human body can be assessed according to laboratory tests of human blood. In this case, blood parameters can be biomarkers of the impact of atmospheric air pollution on the body, which will allow assessing the adverse effects of the factor more quickly and accurately, comparable to the use of incidence rates. Quite widely in the literature are studies of the effect of air pollution on blood counts. Exposure to the particulate matter contained in the atmospheric air can cause a decrease in the content of high-density lipoproteins [19]. Combined exposure to $PM_{2.5}$ and black carbon for 3 months or more causes a decrease in the content of high-density lipoproteins in the blood, more pronounced among the female population [20].

The combined effect of nitrogen dioxide, sulfur dioxide, and carbon monoxide exposure in the air can lead to a decrease in the iron content in the blood serum and to the development of iron deficiency anemia [21]. In China, an increase in blood glucose levels was found with 4 days of exposure to sulfur dioxide, nitrogen dioxide, and PM_{10}, and this effect was more pronounced among women, the elderly, and overweight people [22].

5. Conclusion

Control over the state of atmospheric air in the Republic of Belarus is carried out regularly by the Ministry of Health and the Ministry of Natural Resources and Environmental Protection. Special attention is paid to the content of the main pollutants, specific pollutants (in the area of industrial enterprises), as well as their combinations, which have a proven effect of summation in the joint presence (45 summation groups).

Over the past 20 years, there has been a decrease in both the content of individual pollutants in the atmospheric air and the amount of emissions from stationary and mobile sources, and today, there is almost no excess of national air quality standards for the average annual content of individual pollutants.

Nevertheless, the effects of atmospheric air pollution remain the object of close attention and have been proven to contribute to the formation of the health status of the population. In connection with the foregoing, a promising direction in the policy for the control of atmospheric air pollution in the Republic of Belarus is the assessment of pollution levels according to complex indicators that take into account the entire spectrum of pollution and the fact of simultaneous exposure of a person to a large number of pollutants in concentrations not exceeding the values of hygienic standards. However, the absence of the above complex indicators of legal force at the moment does not allow taking active preventive measures on the basis of these indicators.

Acknowledgements

The authors express their gratitude to the National Statistical Committee of the Republic of Belarus, the Center for Radiation Control and Environmental Monitoring of the Republic of Belarus, and the Ministry of Health of the Republic of Belarus for using their publicly available data.

Conflict of interest

The authors declare no conflict of interest.

Author details

Nadzeya Dziarzhynskaya*, Larisa Hindziuk and Andrey Hindziuk
Belarusian State Medical University, Minsk, Belarus

*Address all correspondence to: klishka@mail.ru

References

[1] Zaitseva NV, May IV, Shur PZ, Kiryanov DA. Methodological approaches for assessment performance and economical efficiency of the risk-oriented control and supervision of the federal service on customers rights protection and human well-being surveillance (Rospotrebnadzor). Health Risk Analysis. 2014;**1**:7-9

[2] WHO (World Health Organization). EUR/RC65/18. 2015. Progress report on the European Environment and Health Process. [Internet]. 2015. Available from: http://www.euro.who.int/__data/assets/pdf_file/0006/283839/65wd18e_EHP_150476.pdf?ua=1 [accessed 01 June 2022].

[3] Filonov VP, Sokolov SM, Naumenko TE. Ecological and Epidemiological Risk Assessment for Human Health of Atmospheric Quality. Minsk: TRANSTEXT; 2001. p. 187

[4] Chebotarev PA, Aprasyuhipa NI, Yaskevich VV, Kozlova LI, Parchinskaya TV, Chebotarev SP. Hygienic assessment of atmospheric air pollution by oil hydrocarbons. Hygiene and Sanitation. 2003;**6**:56-58

[5] Medvedev IV. Environmental Protection: Statistical Collection. Minsk: National Statistical Committee; 2021. p. 202

[6] National Statistical Committee of the Republic of Belarus. Air pollution and ozone depletion. [Internet]. 2022. Available from: https://www.belstat.gov.by/ofitsialnaya-statistika/makroekonomika-i-okruzhayushchaya-sreda/okruzhayuschaya-sreda/sovmestnaya-sistema-ekologicheskoi-informatsii2/a-zagryaznenie-atmosfernogo-vozduha-i-razrushenie-ozonovogo-sloya/

[7] Republican Center for Hydrometeorology, Radioactive Pollution Control and Environmental Monitoring. Radiation and Environmental Monitoring. Atmospheric air monitoring. [Internet]. 2022. Available from: https://rad.org.by/articles/vozduh/monitoring-atmosfernogo-vozduha

[8] National Legal Internet Portal of the Republic of Belarus. Resolution of the Council of Ministers of the Republic of Belarus. On the approval of hygiene standards. [Internet]. 2021. Available from: http://cgevtb.by/files/files/imce/postanovlenie_sov_min_37.pdf.

[9] Gritsenko TD. Ecological and Epidemiological Assessment of the Risk of Atmospheric Pollution for Public Health. Minsk: Minsk State Medical Institute; 2001. p. 21

[10] Dziarzhynskaya N, Hindziuk A, Hindziuk L, Sysoeva I, Krupskaya D, Urban U, et al. Airborne chemical pollution and children's asthma incidence rate in Minsk. Journal of Preventive Medicine and Hygiene. 2021; **62**:E871-E878

[11] Sokolov S. M., Gritsenko T.D., Fedorovich S.V. [et al.] The incidence of allergic rhinitis and asthma in the children's population of Minsk, depending on the qualitative and quantitative composition of aeroallergens in the atmospheric air. Health and Environment: Collection of Materials International Scientific and Practical Conferences. 2018;1:34-36

[12] Sokolov SM, Shevchuk LM, Gankin AN, Pozniak IS. On the issue of assessing the risk to public health of atmospheric air pollution. Vestnik VGMU. 2015;**4**:92-97

[13] Pshegroda AE. Hygienic risk assessment for public health of exposure to carcinogens and toxicants in the atmospheric air. Belarusian Medical Journal. 2004;**4**:84-87

[14] Atkinson RW, Analitis A, Samoli E, Fuller GW, Green DC, Mudway IS, et al. Short-term exposure to traffic-related air pollution and daily mortality in London, UK. Journal of Exposure Science and Environmental Epidemiology. 2016; **26**(2):125-132

[15] Tseng E, Ho WC, Lin MH, Cheng TJ, Chen PC, Lin HH. Chronic exposure to particulate matter and risk of cardiovascular mortality: cohort study from Taiwan. BMC Public Health. 2015; **15**:936

[16] Clancy L, Goodman P, Sinclair H, Dockery DW. Effect of air-pollution control on death rates in Dublin, Ireland: an intervention study. Lancet. 2002; **360**(9341):1210-1214

[17] Männistö T, Mendola P, Laughon Grantz K, Leishear K, Sundaram R, Sherman S, et al. Acute and recent air pollution exposure and cardiovascular events at labour and delivery. Heart. 2015;**101**(18):1491-1498

[18] Chiang TY, Yuan TH, Shie RH, Chen CF, Chan CC. Increased incidence of allergic rhinitis, bronchitis and asthma, in children living near a petrochemical complex with SO_2 pollution. Environment International. 2016 Nov;**96**:1-7

[19] Koman PD, Hogan KA, Sampson N, Mandell R, Coombe CM, Tetteh MM, et al. Examining joint effects of air pollution exposure and social determinants of health in defining "At-Risk" populations under the clean air act: Susceptibility of pregnant women to hypertensive disorders of pregnancy. World Medical & Health Policy. 2018; **10**(1):7-54

[20] Bell G, Mora S, Greenland P, Tsai M, Gill E, Kaufman JD. Association of air pollution exposures with high-density lipoprotein cholesterol and particle number: The multi-ethnic study of atherosclerosis. Arteriosclerosis Thrombosis Vascular Biology. 2017; **37**(5):976-982

[21] Balabina NM. The role of atmospheric air poisoning in the development of iron deficiency anemia in the adult urban population. Hygiene and Sanitation. 2006;**6**:12-14

[22] Chen L, Zhou Y, Li S, Williams G, Kan H, Marks GB, et al. Air pollution and fasting blood glucose: A longitudinal study in China. Science of the Total Environment. 2016;**541**:750-755